Stop Smoking Lose Weight

Also by Dr. Neil Solomon

The Truth About Weight Control
Dr. Solomon's Easy No-Risk Diet
Dr. Solomon's Proven Master Plan for
  Total Body Fitness and Maintenance
Dr. Solomon's High Health Diet and
  Exercise Plan

Stop Smoking Lose Weight

Neil Solomon, M.D., Ph.D.

G. P. Putnam's Sons, New York

Copyright © 1981 by Neil Solomon, M.D., Ph.D.
All rights reserved. This book, or portions thereof,
must not be reproduced in any form without permission.
Published simultaneously in Canada by Academic Press
Canada Limited, Toronto.

Exercise photographs by Alexander Karas

Library of Congress Cataloging in Publication Data

Solomon, Neil, date.
    Stop smoking, lose weight.
       1. Reducing diets. 2. Smoking. 3. Cigarette habit.
I. Title.
RM222.2.S654   613.8'5   81-1519
ISBN 0-399-12600-7   AACR2

PRINTED IN THE UNITED STATES OF AMERICA

I dedicate this book to Mildred Sindell, who is now a successful ex-smoker. Her insight into the problems of giving up cigarettes resulted in many of the tips in this book. Her help with bringing this book to fruition was momentous.

AND

I dedicate this book to my loving, talented, and patient wife, Frema, who is my first choice as wife, mistress, and mother of my children.

Without her, I could not have been blessed with my three wonderful and talented sons, Ted, Scott, and Cliff, who, along with Frema, make me very, very, happy.

AND

I dedicate this book to all my patients who have allowed me to help them and from whom I've learned so very much. I thank you and wish you continued success.

Acknowledgments

It would be difficult to name all the people who so generously contributed their time and effort to this book. Busy members of the medical profession, both researchers and practicing physicians, have unstintingly given of their time and released new data to me. Many others, through their published findings, have also contributed to the fund of knowledge and understanding of the problems of the overweight and smoking patient.

Although I cannot name every individual who contributed to this effort, I would especially like to thank:

Rob Fitz Cressa Goodman
Harry Finkelstein Miriam Glazer
Marion F. Hanna R.D. Beverly Willner
Betye-Lynn Steiner Evalee Harrison
Lynn Rosen Richard Sindell
Mildred Sindell Ro Defeo
Helen Fleischer Peter and Reta Sindell

Dr. Garry Nyman
Frema Solomon
Ted Solomon
Scott Solomon
Cliff Solomon
Francis Rackemann
Betty Coppel
Denise Ayres
Nancy E. Bayne
Timothy B. Johnson
Joyce Parseghian
Terry Hazel
Joe and Joann Mermis
Dr. Neil Pauker
Dr. Fred Berlin

Peter and Reta Sindell
Ann McMath
Leslie Schoenberger
Meryl Latish
Carolyn Bradley
Joan Deuerling
Dr. Roger Palmer
Dr. George Mogil
Ester Newberg
David Finkelstein
Ginette Salvadore
Suellen Poland
Sam Bloom
Bill Nicholson
Bea Weitzel

Author's Note:

Pertinent scientific data used in this book has been published in medical journals, or has been accepted for publication in the *Maryland State Medical Journal*.

I have made a few changes in my patients' case study circumstances in order to prevent any possible identification of, or embarrassment to, them.

Contents

Introduction		11
1	If You Need Convincing	15
2	Current Quitters' Programs	27
3	"Physician, Heal Thyself"	35
4	Breaking Away	39
5	Tensions—How to Hurdle	47
6	Weighing Too Much	53
7	Group Support and Dieting	61
8	A Critique of Other Approaches	69
9	Why *This* Diet?	79
10	My Stop-Smoking, Lose-Weight Diet	85
11	A French Connection	109
12	Stop Smoking in Only One Day?	117
13	Proof of the Pudding	121
14	Slimming Tips	127
Afterword		187

Introduction

Stop smoking and lose weight! Sounds too good to be true, doesn't it? That's what a lot of my patients told me. Many said they were reluctant to stop smoking because they would make up for it by overeating.

By and large, my patients had a valid point. When they stopped smoking, the majority of them did gain weight. I was trying to find a solution for what up until now seemed an insoluble problem.

Over the years I have been devising sensible, nutritionally balanced, weight-loss diets. These diets work well for people who want to lose weight and keep it off permanently (*Dr. Solomon's Easy, No-Risk Diet*). However, patients who give up smoking have the additional problem of craving nicotine at the time of withdrawal.

I kept thinking whether through food there was any chemical interaction that might help lessen the patients' craving for nicotine. Thus, I developed the Stop-Smoking, Lose-Weight Diet.

This diet, because of the increased chemical alkalinity it provides, allows nicotine to slowly leave the body, thus lessening craving and at the same time cutting down on calories. So, America, if you want to stop smoking and lose weight, this is the book for you.

The American people, battered by constant warnings about the variety of environmental substances harmful to their health, have had their senses somewhat dulled. Yet, these warnings should not be taken lightly. We may joke all we want about the "carcinogen-of-the-day," just so long as we accept and heed the seriousness of the message.

Many of us react to the flurry of warnings about real and imagined dangers to health by developing a "What's-the-use?" attitude. If everything is hazardous, some argue, we may as well enjoy life fully without worrying about potential dangers that lurk in every corner. As suggested in Isaiah, "Let us eat and drink; for tomorrow we shall die."

The fallacy in this type of reasoning is that no one claims that *everything* is hazardous. Everyone sincerely interested in promoting good health has the capacity to do something about it. In many instances it is not fate that accounts for our susceptibility to disease and even death, but life-style.

One study has shown that adherence to just seven habits can have a significant effect on a person's health. They include eating moderately, eating regularly, eating breakfast, no cigarette smoking, exercise, moderate or no use of alcohol, and seven to eight hours sleep each night.

The study showed that a forty-five-year-old man who adhered to just three or four of these habits could look forward to twenty-two more years of life. For those who followed four to five or six to seven of the habits, the additional expected longevity would be twenty-eight and thirty-three years, respectively.

The importance of life-style on our health and well-being is further highlighted by Dr. Lester Breslow of the University of California, Los Angeles. He notes that blacks in this country show significantly higher total death rates, infant deaths, and death from lung cancer and acts of violence than do whites. On the other hand, Japanese-Americans enjoy better health than either whites or blacks, and Mormons have a 25 to 40 percent lower mortality rate than whites of other religious persuasions.

These differences cannot be attributed to race or religion as such, or even to luck; rather, they stem from one's lifestyle, and the question we should ponder is: What is there about the way the Japanese or Mormons live that accounts for their lower death rate?

One factor accounting for differences in health between populations is diet. For example, studies reveal that Japanese have a lower incidence of cancer of the colon than Americans. However, Japanese who emigrate to the United States eventually assume the health characteristics of their new land. It is believed that differences in diet may in large part account for this.

Further evidence that to a great extent we are masters of our own fate is contained in statistics reflecting the adverse effects of increased cigarette smoking among the people of developing nations. According to Drs. Phyllis Piotrow and Samuel Ward of the Johns Hopkins School of Hygiene and Public Health, greater cigarette consumption among childbearing women in these countries is already taking a significant toll. In Dacca, Bangladesh, for example, twice as many babies born to nonsmokers survived than those born to smokers. These infants died either before or shortly after birth.

The important point is that we are not helpless in the face of threats to our health. A great deal of illness and even death result simply because we abuse or neglect our bodies. Neither smoking nor obesity, for example, is beyond our ability to control.

A poll by the Louis Harris Company of more than 1,500 people showed that 67 percent believed they would be healthier if they changed their eating habits; 62 percent said they knew they should get more exercise; and an equal number of people who were overweight said they knew the added pounds were bad for them.

While no one can guarantee that a person will not have a heart attack or a variety of other diseases, the risks can be reduced. Most people seriously interested in curbing their smoking and losing weight at the same time will find the means of doing so in this book.

1 • If You Need Convincing

A visitor from another planet undoubtedly would find a number of mind-boggling situations to contemplate, but none more so than this country's attitude towards smoking. How could we explain to an alien guest that while one segment of the United States government is busily spreading the word about the ravages of death and disease attributable to cigarette smoking, another department of the same government is using taxpayers' money to subsidize farmers who grow tobacco?

And how would we explain that although nine of every ten cigarette smokers, apparently aware of the hazards, profess a desire to quit smoking, the production and consumption of cigarettes are at an all-time high? In fact, such contradictory, self-defeating behavior is difficult to explain even to ourselves.

Tobacco is a major agricultural crop in the United States, and any effort to restrict its cultivation would have far-reaching social, economic, and political reverberations. Yet even the tobacco industry, despite periodic denials of an association between cigarette smoking and a variety of diseases, is seeking to develop a product containing less tar and nicotine, and advertises strongly and widely those cigarettes with lowest amounts of these substances.

The surgeon general of the United States has termed cigarette smoking "the single most important preventable environmental factor contributing to illness, disability, and death in the United States." Of the approximately 100,000 deaths from lung cancer in this country in 1980, from 85 to 90 percent were traceable to smoking.

Moreover, cigarette smokers are at a demonstrably increased risk of developing cancer of the larynx, pharynx, oral cavity, esophagus, pancreas, kidney, and bladder.

Smoking affects the body in various ways. In the 1979 *Surgeon General's Report*, we see . . . "Smoking of tobacco should be considered as one of the primary sources of drug interactions in man." For example, the effectiveness of vaccinations may be compromised if a person smokes. Vaccines stimulate the development of antibodies, which protect the body against disease. Research suggests that influenza vaccine, for example, produces many fewer antibodies in smokers than in nonsmokers.

A smoking-nutrition interaction is another possible hazard. Smoking changes the way the body metabolizes carbohydrates and proteins. In addition, smokers seem to have an increased need for vitamin C. This may account for the greater bone mineral loss found in postmenopausal women who smoke than in postmenopausal women who do not smoke.

The hazards of smoking are well-documented. The director of surgical research at the University of Chicago,

Dr. A. R. Mossa, has warned that cigarette smokers have the greatest risk of developing lung cancer. But, he adds, if lung cancer doesn't get you, pancreatic cancer very well may. And Dr. J. Patterson Browder, assistant professor of surgery at the University of North Carolina, says: "I can't recall having seen a patient with cancer of the larynx in the last five years who was not a heavy smoker." In all, cigarette smoking is a major factor in about 345,000 deaths each year from cancer and diseases of the heart, lungs, and circulatory system.

Further evidence of the association between cigarette smoking and lung cancer is seen in the recent increased incidence of the disease in women. During the past thirty years—a period marked by a substantial increase in smoking among women—their lung cancer rate rose 400 percent. It is estimated that if the trend continues, by 1983 lung cancer will have replaced breast cancer as the leading cause of death from cancer in women.

Women who smoke are five times as likely to get lung cancer as those who do not smoke, and twice as prone to get bladder cancer as light smokers or nonsmokers, according to data gathered by the American Medical Association's Educational Research Foundation. Moreover, women who use alcohol *and* smoke cigarettes are at greater risk from tongue, esophageal, and mouth cancer.

One well-publicized problem is the increased risk of heart attack, stroke, and other circulatory diseases among women who smoke and use oral contraceptives. This has led many physicians to warn their patients that they should not smoke if they use oral contraceptives, or, conversely, not to use oral contraceptives if they smoke.

The 1980 *Surgeon General's Report to Congress on Smoking* notes that in 1968 women accounted for one in six fatal cases of cancer; today the figure has increased to one in four. Apparently, women are no less susceptible to the effects of smoking cigarettes—as was once believed—than are men.

Nor can nonsmokers who live, work, or come into contact with smokers breathe easily, secure in the knowledge that their abstinence protects them from the dangers of smoking. There is substantial evidence implicating passive or involuntary smoking—that is, the inhalation of tobacco smoke by a nonsmoker—as a risk factor in cancer and heart disease. A study conducted at Edinboro State College in Pennsylvania revealed that: "Nonsmoking wives whose husbands did not smoke cigarettes lived four years longer than those whose husbands smoked cigarettes."

The list of those at risk from cigarette smoke still is not complete. Another group consists of those still unborn. Infants whose mothers smoked during their pregnancies are more likely to be of low birth weight and have a greater chance of dying soon after birth than babies born to nonsmoking mothers. In addition, women who smoke while pregnant show a greater incidence of stillbirths, spontaneous abortions, and premature deliveries. Other effects may include impaired physical and emotional development.

A study by the Office on Smoking and Health of the former Department of Health, Education, and Welfare (HEW) summarizes the relationship between smoking and overall deaths as follows:

- Overall death rates for cigarette smokers are about 70 percent higher than those for nonsmokers.

- Overall death risk increases with the amount smoked. For the two-pack-a-day cigarette smoker, the risk of premature death is approximately twice that of the nonsmoker.

- Overall death ratios of smokers compared to nonsmokers are highest at earlier ages and decline with increasing age. For cigarette smokers, the risk of premature death is twice that of nonsmokers at age forty.

- Overall death ratios are higher for those who begin smoking at a young age compared to those who begin later. For those who begin smoking before the age of fifteen, the risk of premature death is about 86 percent higher than that for nonsmokers.

- Overall death ratios are higher for those smokers who inhale than for those who do not.

- There is about a 15 percent reduction in overall death risk for smokers of low-"tar" and nicotine cigarettes (less than 17.6 mg. "tar" and less than 1.2 mg. nicotine) compared to those who smoke high "tar" and nicotine cigarettes (25.8–35.7 mg. "tar" and 2.0–2.7 mg. nicotine).

However, overall death rates of low "tar" and nicotine cigarette smokers are still about 50 percent higher than for nonsmokers.

This may give us a clue. In one study conducted by Dr. Stanley Schachter, participants alternated between smoking high/low nicotine cigarettes; without exception, long-time heavy smokers consumed more of the low-nicotine cigarettes, with an average increase in smoking of 25 percent. Even though heavy smokers as a group expressed an intense dislike for the low-nicotine cigarettes, they smoked a far larger number than of the high-nicotine cigarettes, which they found acceptable.

The study suggests that heavy smokers who switch to low-nicotine brands of cigarettes not only regulate their smoking so as to obtain the same amounts of nicotine and tar as with the high-nicotine brands, but subject themselves to more of the products of combustion, such as carbon monoxide, as well.

The same *HEW Report* has this to say on the death rates for pipe and cigar smokers:

- Overall death ratios for cigar smokers are somewhat higher than for nonsmokers. The *U. S. Veterans Study* showed a death ratio of 1.16, compared to 1.0 for nonsmokers. The overall death ratio was 39 percent higher than the ratio in nonsmokers for men smoking nine or more cigars a day. A positive dose-response relationship exists between cigar smoking and deaths.

- Overall death ratios for male cigar smokers are inversely proportional to the age at which the individual began smoking.

- Overall death ratios for pipe smokers are only slightly higher than for nonsmokers. The death ratio in the *U. S. Veterans Study* was 1.07. Overall death ratios were 21 percent higher than nonsmokers for men who smoked twenty or more pipefuls a day than for nonsmokers. A positive dose-response relationship exists between pipe smoking and deaths.

- Overall death ratios of men who smoke cigarettes in combination with pipes and/or cigars are intermediate between those who smoke pipes or cigars only and those who smoke cigarettes only. Cigarette smokers who also smoke cigars or pipes have overall death rates approximately 30 percent higher than nonsmokers.

The death figures start looking better for former smokers.

- Overall death rates of former smokers decline as the

number of years of cessation increase. After fifteen years off cigarettes, death rates for former smokers are nearly identical to those of nonsmokers.

- Overall death rates of former smokers are directly proportional to the number of cigarettes the person used to smoke.

- Overall death rates of former smokers are inversely proportional to the age at which the person began smoking.

- Regardless of length of time smoked or number of cigarettes smoked, former smokers have lower death rates than continuing smokers, provided they are not ill at the time of cessation.

Dr. John Holbrook, of the University of Utah Medical School, writing in Harrison's *Principles of Internal Medicine*, looked into large prospective studies of populations in various countries. The chief contributor to the excess death rate in male smokers is coronary heart disease, which accounts for more than twice as many deaths as lung cancer, the second leading cause. In general, the risk of coronary heart disease is 60 percent to 70 percent greater in men who smoke than in those who do not. On the other hand, those who stop smoking decrease their risk of death from coronary heart disease, an effect that becomes measurable within one year after quitting.

Moreover, people who continue to smoke after an acute myocardial infarction are more likely to die from coronary heart disease than those who stop. In addition, cigarette smokers in the United States suffer more disability as a result of chronic illness, and have an absentee work record 45 percent greater than do nonsmokers.

The added risk of a smoker developing lung cancer is also well documented. Men who smoke a pack of cigarettes a day have ten times the risk of getting the disease as do nonsmokers; and those who smoke two packs a day may have twenty-five times the risk.

As if this weren't sufficiently threatening, workers in certain industries who also smoke are at especially high risk for lung cancer. The ability of two substances to combine to produce an effect that either one alone is not capable of is called "synergism." Thus, people who work in the asbestos or uranium mining industries—which in themselves are high-risk occupations—and who, in addition, smoke, are playing a form of Russian roulette in which almost all the chambers of the gun carry a live cartridge.

Cigarette smoking also contributes to the development of chronic obstructive pulmonary disease—that is, chronic bronchitis and emphysema. Approximately 70 percent of the 25,000 deaths from this cause in the United States in 1978 were attributable to smoking, and many of these deaths followed prolonged periods of respiratory disability.

According to Dr. Holbrook, men who smoke cigarettes suffer from four to twenty-five times the number of deaths from chronic obstructive pulmonary disease than do nonsmokers. For most people in the United States, smoking is a more important cause of the condition than occupational or environmental factors. Here, too, those who stop smoking show a decrease in mortality from chronic obstructive pulmonary disease, a decrease in pulmonary symptoms, and improved pulmonary function.

That smoking has these effects is not surprising. As much as 90 percent of cigarette smoke consists of gases that are hazardous to health; the remainder, particulate matter, includes nicotine, which is the addictive element in tobacco, and tar.

Carbon monoxide makes up from one to five percent of cigarette smoke; when inhaled, that compound displaces oxygen in the blood, forming carboxyhemoglobin. In the smoker, this chemical reaction increases hardening of the arteries and leads to disease of the respiratory system and to sudden death from coronary heart disease.

In case you wonder about substituting snuff or chewing tobacco for cigarettes, read on. The use of snuff or chewing tobacco as a means of breaking the cigarette habit may be a case of going from the frying pan into the fire. An article in the *Journal of the American Medical Association* by Dr. Alan Blum indicates that the use of chewing tobacco and snuff may be more dangerous to health in some respects than smoking cigarettes. He notes that snuff can cause gum disease, tooth abrasion, and cancer of the throat, while chewing tobacco may lead to cancer of the mouth, throat, and digestive tract. His conclusions were based on a number of studies by medical researchers, including one of more than 2,000 subjects in India who used chewing tobacco.

With all this mounting evidence as to why people should *not* smoke, one may wonder why so many do. Given the well-established association between cigarette smoking and a host of diseases, it must be assumed that except for smokers with a well-developed self-destructive urge, most would prefer to kick the habit but are too strongly addicted to do so. In other words, continued smoking is not so much an indication of a person's unwillingness to stop smoking, as of an inability to stop.

The National Cancer Institute suggests that several motives are responsible for the continued smoking by fifty-four million people in the United States. The reasons given include: (1) a sense of increased energy or stimulation; (2) the satisfaction of handling or manipulating things; (3) the accentuation of pleasure and relaxation; (4) the reduction of negative feelings such as anxiety and anger; (5) craving or psychological addiction; and (6) habit.

For many people smoking serves as a psychological crutch, easing nervous tension while providing oral gratification. Some health professionals attribute the increased smoking by women to the stresses confronting them as a result of feeling they have to be "superwomen"—all things to all people, juggling their own lives as well as those around them, while staying in control and functioning well in all areas. Regardless of the reason, women are rapidly achieving equality with men in the incidence of smoking-related diseases.

The National Cancer Institute notes further that: "The majority of current smokers have made a serious attempt to stop smoking at least once, or say they would do so if there were any easy way to quit. Most smokers have also tried to cut down the number of cigarettes they smoke each day without trying to stop smoking entirely."

All this suggests that most smokers are aware of the health hazards of their habit and would welcome a cure that is simple, effective, painless, free of significant adverse side effects, and inexpensive. Until now, however, this seemed an unrealistic and unattainable goal.

Whereas some diseases, such as cancer of the lung, that are attributable to cigarette smoking may take up to twenty or more years to develop, the benefits of quitting become apparent much more quickly. The National Institutes of Health (NIH) notes that the body begins to heal itself within twelve hours after a person stops smoking. Among the immediate health benefits is a rapid decline in the carbon monoxide level in the blood. As the level decreases, the heart and lungs begin to repair the damage caused by the cigarette smoke.

While smoking causes a person to feel tired and lethargic, draining away energy and stamina, giving up cigarettes helps restore vigor and strength. The ex-smoker breathes more easily and does not become winded so readily.

While smoking produces a foul taste in the mouth, giving up cigarettes restores the sense of taste and clean breath. Eating becomes more enjoyable, food tastes better, and the digestive system begins to return to normal.

While smoking often results in headaches, sensations of dizziness, and a hacking cough, giving up cigarettes helps restore the ex-smoker's sense of well-being. Gone is the smoker's hack as well as the headaches and dizzy spells caused by the cigarettes.

Almost as important, the mess, smell, inconvenience, expense, and dependence associated with cigarette smoking becomes a thing of the past.

The long-range benefits of giving up cigarettes are even more significant:

- After ten to fifteen years without cigarettes, the risk of premature death for ex-smokers approaches that for people who never smoked.

- After ten to fifteen years without cigarettes, the risk of lung cancer approaches that for people who never smoked.

- After ten years, the risk of cancer of the larynx is the same as that for people who never smoked.

- After ten to fifteen years, the risk of mouth cancer is the same as that for people who never smoked.

- After seven years, the risk of bladder cancer is the same as that for people who never smoked.

- And after ten years, the risk of coronary heart disease is the same as that for people who never smoked.

Any one of these reasons should be sufficient to turn a smoker into an ex-smoker. Taken together, the reasons for giving up cigarettes are overwhelming.

According to NIH, one of every five days a smoker misses from work because of illness is attributable to smoking, as is one in every ten days a smoker is confined to bed because of an illness.

The ex-smoker, on the other hand, not only can look forward to a longer life, but to a happier and more productive one as well.

So how successful you will be in reducing the number of cigarettes smoked or in quitting seems governed by a number of things: how much smoking maintains your psychological equilibrium, how concerned you are about what smoking is doing to your health, and how much true control you have over your behavior. All of these must be reinforced by your belief that stopping will help you in the long run.

It's up to you.

2 • Current Quitters' Programs

Recognition of the hazards of smoking, to smokers and nonsmokers alike, has resulted in a proliferation of programs designed to help people kick the habit. But while some individuals undoubtedly have been helped to quit, statistics indicate that conventional approaches to the problem are not very successful.

The National Cancer Institute notes that 90 percent of the fifty-four million Americans who smoke want to give it up, but are unable to do so. Sixty percent have tried unsuccessfully to stop, and an additional 30 percent say they would try if there were an easy way to do so. Smokers are concerned about their health, but many are too addicted to nicotine to do anything constructive about it.

In light of this perceived need for assistance, it is no wonder that a variety of smoking-cessation programs have flourished in recent years. Despite their prevalence, however, only two percent of smokers who want to quit have been sufficiently motivated to attend formal stop-smoking clinics.

In attempting to devise a solution to this widespread problem, we should bear in mind that smoking provides the habituated person with some form of satisfaction—physiological, psychological, or social. Smokers develop a strong addiction to the nicotine in tobacco, a substance that can act as a stimulant, depressant, or tranquilizer, depending on the dosage.

For many people, even efforts to reduce the hazards of smoking by switching to low-tar and nicotine cigarettes are doomed to failure. The smoker who really is hooked will unconsciously consume cigarettes at a rate that provides the level of nicotine required by the brain to produce the desired effect. This is accomplished either by inhaling more deeply, smoking more cigarettes, or smoking more of each cigarette. Nicotine is absorbed from the lungs almost immediately after the tobacco smoke is inhaled. Pipe or cigar-smoking and chewing tobacco provide a slower rate of absorption.

The best way to deal with smoking obviously is never to start. Very few people are occasional smokers; once they start, most become regularly dependent on the habit.

Programs to curb smoking are offered under a variety of auspices and employ a variety of approaches. These include individual and group therapy, hypnosis, acupuncture, pharmaceutical aids, and aversion techniques, a form of behavior modification. In fact, behavior modification is used as an adjunct form of treatment with many other methods.

The pharmaceuticals used in these programs include products designed to serve as a substitute for tobacco, such as nicotine chewing gum; deterrents, such as astringent mouthwashes, which irritate the oral and nasal mucosa;

and medications that have a relaxing effect, thus reducing the physiological and psychological withdrawal symptoms associated with attempts to stop smoking.

The more common aversion techniques include rapid smoking, a method that requires the subject to inhale rapidly until additional smoking becomes intolerable, and electric shock. The National Cancer Institute notes that rapid smoking poses a danger, and suggests it be used only under close medical supervision so that anyone who experiences a cardiac emergency can receive appropriate treatment. Reports indicate that electric shock when used alone has not been very effective.

Another aversive technique, similar to but different from rapid smoking, is satiation. Rather than increasing the rate at which cigarettes are smoked, the subject increases the number smoked. As with rapid smoking satiation is best done under medical supervision since it results in high levels of nicotine which could adversely affect the cardiopulmonary system.

Other programs try to frighten smokers into giving up the habit by showing films graphically depicting lung diseases and associated surgery, emphasizing statistics on disease and death attributable to smoking, and lecturing on its dangers. While the success of these efforts is difficult to assess with any real degree of accuracy, the data suggest they have made no significant impact in resolving a problem that literally is a matter of life and death.

Group therapy programs are sponsored in a number of communities by nonprofit agencies, including local chapters of national health organizations such as the American Cancer Society, the American Heart Association, and the American Lung Association, as well as by commercial enterprises. The group leader may be a psychiatrist, psychologist, social worker, or other professional. The aim of these programs is to help participants understand why they smoke and how they can give it up, an effort in which each member is supported by the group as a whole.

One of the better known commercial group therapy programs is conducted by SmokEnders. According to the literature it distributes, participants meet for about two hours a week. During the first five weeks, smokers are encouraged to continue smoking as in the past. After the fifth meeting, however, they are supposed to be physically and psychologically prepared to quit.

After this point, the program continues for four more weeks, during which time the now ex-smoker is helped to adjust. "When the program is over," SmokEnders notes, "you are a comfortable nonsmoker on the way to a new, healthier, happier, life."

The Seventh-Day Adventist Church sponsors a "5-Day Plan to Stop Smoking." It claims to show "how to beat the smoking habit on all four dimensions of life, physical, mental, social, and spiritual." Sessions usually are conducted jointly by a Seventh-Day Adventist physician and a clergyman, and include talks, films, and group discussion.

The "5-Day Plan" advocates a cold-turkey approach, explaining: "It is better to have a few rough days and be through with it than to drag it out for weeks and months. Slow torture is no fun."

To support the participant's resolve to quit, Dr. J. Wayne McFarland, co-developer of the "Plan," suggests the following: (1) a warm bath two or three times a day; (2) drinking six to eight glasses of water a day—but no alcoholic beverages, tea, coffee, or cola drinks—to help remove the nicotine from the system; (3) regular times for meals and adequate rest; (4) walking, rather than sitting around, after meals; (5) avoidance of highly spiced foods, rich or greasy fried foods, and rich desserts; (6) eating freely of fruits, vegetables, grains, and nuts; (7) use of wheat germ or dried brewer's yeast; (8) a mild tranquilizer, but only with a physician's approval; and (9) praying for divine help.

Another smoking cessation program is offered by Schick Laboratories, a commercial organization. It stresses behavior modification and aversion therapy within a framework of five one-hour individual sessions. The approach includes rapid smoking and electric shock applied to the arm. Eight one-hour group meetings, which include films and lectures, reinforce the individual therapy sessions.

A number of organizations employ hypnosis, either alone or in combination with other techniques, to help participants stop smoking. In some programs, an effort is made to have the subject associate smoking with unpleasant thoughts, making it essentially an aversion technique. In general, reports about the effectiveness of hypnosis in getting people to stop smoking are contradictory. There is some agreement, however, that the success of the technique is enhanced when combined with other approaches, such as individual or group therapy.

Both the National Cancer Institute and the American Cancer Society publish booklets which, in effect, are do-it-yourself guides to stop smoking. Many of their suggestions involve behavior modification techniques—for example, "If you miss the sensation of having a cigarette in your hand, play with something else—a pencil, a paper clip, a marble." And "If you miss having something in your mouth, try toothpicks or a fake cigarette."

Smokers trying to break the habit are instructed to drink lots of water; to nibble on fruit, celery, carrots, and cookies; or to take a candy mint or chewing gum when the desire for a cigarette increases. At the end of a meal, a mouthwash rather than a cigarette is recommended. Finally, the smoker who has become an ex-smoker is urged to enjoy a deserved reward by purchasing something with the money that otherwise would have been spent on cigarettes.

Some desperate smokers have even turned to smokeless cigarettes in an effort to kick the habit. These "cigarettes" contain nicotine but no tobacco. Puffing or inhaling on them, according to Dr. Norman L. Jacobson of San Antonio, gives users the satisfaction they are seeking without the carbon monoxide and tar they would be breathing were they smoking ordinary cigarettes.

Each smokeless cigarette provides about one-half the nicotine delivered by a conventional puff, and it can be used all day. However, the smokeless cigarettes do have drawbacks. Adverse side effects include faintness, hiccups, and nausea.

One of the more comprehensive surveys of stop-smoking programs was sponsored by the Center for Disease Control (CDC) of the United States Public Health Service. In *Review and Evaluation of Smoking Control Methods: The United States and Canada, 1969–1977,* the authors, Dr. Jerome L. Schwartz and Gail Rider, note that: "From World War I's mass introduction of tobacco to the American Public until the 1964 *Surgeon General's Report,* cigarette use was never questioned publicly." Later, from 1967 to 1971, there was a decrease in the per capita consumption of cigarettes, to some extent because of antismoking advertisements.

Before cigarette advertising on radio and television was prohibited, the equal time provisions of the Federal Communications Act required networks to carry antismoking commercials. Apparently, these public service commercials were extremely effective. Since the ban on cigarette commercials on radio and television, advertising in newspapers and magazines has increased considerably.

One phenomenon of the decade of the '70s was the emergence of antismoking activists—groups such as Action on Smoking and Health (ASH) and Group Against Smoker's Pollution (GASP)—who championed the rights of nonsmokers to a pollution-free environment. As new evidence revealed the dangers inherent in secondhand, or passive, smoking, the lobbying efforts of these organizations assumed a new intensity. Among their goals, some of which have already been achieved, are enactment of legislation restricting smoking in public places—buildings, airplanes, trains, and buses. Many private business establishments and public buildings now have smoking areas set aside, with smoking prohibited in other areas.

Although tobacco company spokespersons for the most part continue to deny any association between smoking and a variety of diseases, tobacco manufacturers have accelerated their efforts to produce low-tar and nicotine cigarettes. A great deal of their advertising, in fact, emphasizes this particular feature more than any other.

Yet, despite the publicity and educational activities, despite the work of advocacy groups, and despite the almost universal acknowledgment by health professionals of smoking's adverse effects, fifty-four million people continue to puff away.

The CDC study cites a report by D. Horn and S. Waingrow, entitled *Some Dimensions of a Model for Smoking Behavior Change,* that lists four aspects of a model for smoking cessation. They include (1) motivation for change; (2) perception of the threat; (3) development and use of alternative psychological mechanisms; and (4) factors facilitating or inhibiting continuing reinforcement.

The perception of the threat requires an awareness and acceptance of the threat, its relevance to the smoker, and his or her susceptibility to intervention. Although it would be difficult to imagine that smokers today are not aware of the threat, many apparently do not acknowledge it or consider it irrelevant. Probably most important, many smokers are not susceptible to intervention.

Until now, no single stop-smoking method applicable to large numbers of people has been developed. To a large extent this reflects the intense addiction to which cigarette smokers are subject. Additionally, however, it should be borne in mind that different people have different smoking habits, they smoke for different reasons, they differ in the extent of their addiction to cigarettes, and—probably of greatest significance—they differ in their determination to break the habit.

Many stop-smoking programs emphasize motivation, determination, and willpower—all important considerations. Others stress smoking's adverse health effects—also a serious consideration. But smoking, like drug or alcohol abuse, is also an addictive habit with physiological ramifications. For a stop-smoking technique to be effective, it must deal with the nicotine in the system as well as the thoughts in the mind.

As for the bottom line, the National Cancer Institute notes that: "A number of evaluation studies by experts in the field of smoking cessation have concluded that no specific technique or program achieves outstanding success." Regardless of the approach, the rate of success—or lack of it—apparently differs little from one method to another.

Meanwhile, fifty-four million Americans continue to smoke.

3 • "Physician, Heal Thyself"

Doctors have taken the biblical injunction "Physician, heal thyself" to heart, at least in relation to smoking. A 1975 study authorized by the Center for Disease Control (CDC) shows that of four groups of health professionals studied—physicians, dentists, pharmacists, and nurses—"Physicians have been the leaders in giving up smoking." The survey found that 55 percent of doctors who previously smoked had not done so for at least ten years, compared with 50 percent of dentists, 47 percent of pharmacists, and 43 percent of nurses.

That large numbers of health professionals have stopped smoking has ramifications far beyond the beneficial effects on their own health. Many people look to their doctors and dentists for guidance in health-related matters, and their advice would be tainted if their actions did not match their words.

The CDC-sponsored study began by obtaining a random sample of about 5,000 names from each of four professional associations—the American Medical Association, the American Dental Association, the American Nurses Association, Inc., and the American Pharmaceutical Association. Since the same groups had been studied a few years earlier (between the spring of 1967 and the summer of 1969), the findings of the two periods could be compared.

The health professionals' responses to the questionnaires they received, or, in some cases to telephone contacts, showed that smoking had decreased substantially since the earlier survey in three of the four groups. Only among nurses had the proportion of those who smoked increased slightly.

Comparing these figures with the incidence of smoking among the general population produced some interesting findings. A national probability sample of adults who smoked showed that the proportion of smokers in each of the three predominantly male health professional groups—doctors, dentists, and pharmacists—was much lower than that of men in the general population, while the proportion of nurses who smoked was higher than among women in the general population.

Smokers among the doctors, dentists, and pharmacists consumed fewer cigarettes and tended to smoke cigarettes lower in tar and nicotine than did men in the general population. On the other hand, there was little difference in the number of cigarettes smoked between nurses and women in the general population, although nurses tended to smoke more low-tar cigarettes.

Most of the health professionals who continued to smoke had started before the association between smoking and disease had become so well known; a majority had made at least one attempt to stop.

As would be expected, health professionals were well aware of the effects of cigarette smoking on health. In fact, 90 percent of the physicians and dentists reported that smoking is a major or contributing cause of lung cancer, chronic bronchitis, emphysema, heart disease, and oral cancer. Between 80 and 90 percent of nurses and pharmacists agreed.

The recognition by physicians of smoking as a serious health hazard is clearly reflected in their treatment of the subject in medical textbooks. In Harrison's *Principles of Internal Medicine,* Dr. John H. Holbrook notes the strong association between cigarette smoking and various diseases. The identification of more than 2,000 substances in cigarette smoke provides a framework for understanding its diverse biologic effects.

Dr. Holbrook divides cigarette smoke into mainstream smoke, which comes out of the mouthpiece when a person is puffing, and sidestream smoke, which is produced at the burning cone and from the mouthpiece between puffs. The composition of the smoke depends on the type of tobacco being burned, the temperature of combustion (which may vary from 30 degrees centigrade at the mouthpiece to 900 degrees centigrade at the burning cone), the length of the cigarette, porosity of the paper, additives, and filter.

Up to 500 milligrams of mainstream smoke—92 percent in a gas phase, and eight percent in a particulate phase—are generated by each cigarette. Mainstream smoke contains two to five billion particles per milliliter!

In addition to nicotine and tar, cigarette smoke in the particulate phase consists of polynuclear aromatic hydrocarbons, phenol, cresol, and trace metals, all of which are carcinogens, plus a number of other substances that also cause cancer or are tumor accelerators. During the gas phase, cigarette smoke consists of these carcinogens: nitrosamines and hydrazine; and these irritants: carbon monoxide, ammonia, and formaldehyde. Some of these constituents of smoke are absorbed through the inner linings of the mouth, nose, pharynx, and upper airways; others are inhaled into the lungs where they are absorbed and retained.

It's known that nicotine is a component of many insecticides. While these poisons do the job on bugs rapidly and efficiently, one should bear in mind that many of the same deleterious effects, albeit at a slower pace, are making themselves felt in humans.

Approximately 50 milligrams of pure nicotine, the amount contained in two cigarettes, are considered sufficient to cause death in humans. The reason a smoker does not die after two cigarettes is that most of the nicotine in cigarettes is burned. Nevertheless, even small amounts of nicotine can cause nausea, vomiting, diarrhea, headaches, dizziness, and high blood pressure, as well as a number of neurological symptoms. Larger doses may result in convulsions, heart irregularities, coma, and the heart suddenly stopping, while still larger amounts can lead to death from lung failure within a matter of a few minutes.

As we learn more and more about the deleterious effects of smoking, an increasing number of health professionals should become better role models for those of us who need all the help we can get to stop.

4 • Breaking Away

You've decided you want to quit smoking. Right? That's great. Let's discuss, openly and honestly, what lies ahead—what pitfalls you might encounter and what rewards you might look forward to.

Over the past two years I have worked intensively with patients who smoked. Many were unsure but hopeful that they could quit. They came confessing that they had tried time and time again to give up smoking, but had been unsuccessful; however, they were willing to try once more. Through them I learned about the strong barriers to quitting—about withdrawal aches and pains. What they shared with me, I shall share with you.

Success in giving up cigarettes and a person's motivation to do so are strongly related. I want you to become aware of what can happen to heavy smokers, both physiologically and psychologically; and when you finally quit, besides offering some good advice and reinforcing tips, I'll suggest emotional supports and substitutions that will help you become successful ex-smokers.

Let's start. You already know that it won't be easy to stop smoking. You will need willpower, lots of it. Why do millions of people continue to smoke even though non-smokers enjoy better health and longer life? Apparently, fear of lingering death from cancer, heart disease, or stroke is not a sufficient deterrent.

Try to think about yourself objectively. I tell my obese patients to stand in front of a mirror in the nude, and to take a good hard look at themselves. They soon begin to realize what they have to do.

The same holds true for smokers. If you've been a heavy smoker, inhale critically for a whiff of your clothes, your hair, your closets, the rooms in your home, your office. You may be surprised how tobacco permeates so much of your life.

Now listen to yourself. How is your breathing? Can you hear a little wheeze? Do you get short of breath climbing stairs or a hill? What about coughing, the hacking kind or spasms? Do you suffer from either?

Many of my patients were so accustomed to these symptoms that they accepted them as a normal, inconvenient part of daily living. Yet once a person stops smoking, these symptoms can improve, even disappear.

Is your breathing shallow? "Each inhaled puff of cigarette smoke delivers a dose of drug to the brain, resulting in 50,000 to 70,000 such doses per person per year. There is no other form of drug taking that occurs with such regularity and frequency." So says the *American Cancer Society Journal,* Autumn, 1980.

We tend to be great deniers. Many of my patients didn't seem to connect their diminished capacity to breathe deeply with the damage caused by the tar and nicotine and carbon monoxide and other substances they had been inhaling for so long. Sure, they have sore throats and other throat illness. But they said, "So what?"

It is encouraging to know that when you do quit smoking, you'll soon see positive results in your pulmonary (lung) function test, and that you'll have less bronchial irritation.

It is also encouraging to read the data on the diminished risk of heart disease for nonsmokers. In fact, three years after quitting, former smokers are no more prone to heart disease than the nonsmokers in the population, and ten years after giving up smoking, ex-smokers have no more chance of suffering lung cancer than people who have never smoked.

Today many public buildings have NO SMOKING signs posted prominently. With increasing frequency we see notices in hospitals, offices, and other public places requesting visitors not to smoke. Railroads, restaurants, and airlines have also cut down on space designed specifically for smokers.

These restrictions against smoking are helpful to the new nonsmoker. They help reduce temptation. It isn't easy to be deprived of the comfort and pleasure many people get from smoking.

"How can I possibly throw away my cigarettes, my crutch that calms me down, eases my tensions, but picks me up so beautifully when I need it?" Ask my patients.

Going cold turkey, I am convinced, is the best way to kick the habit. With gradual withdrawal, a person tends to be jittery, anxious, and angry, while waiting impatiently for the next cigarette.

Be strong. Throw away your cigarettes, ruthlessly. Check all the places where you ordinarily keep or have hidden them. Some of my patients told me that they had them in the refrigerator, freezer, special drawers, and in a tucked away cigarette box. If you are a woman, check each purse for cigarettes and discard them.

Give away or hide all your smoking paraphernalia. Don't even have matches lying around. Stash away the ash trays and lighters. It's too easy to look longingly at these smoking reminders and to start feeling sorry that they are not being used.

This is one time that you've got to grit your teeth, fight the jitters. Because you may very well have them, along with stomach aches and other assorted symptoms.

Regular exercise can be a real lifesaver during this time when you want—you think you need—a cigarette desperately. You can't hold a smoke when you are hitting a golf ball or rolling a bowling ball. Try walking briskly, swinging your arms, or jogging. Utilizing energy this way generally results in a slimmer and firmer body. You don't even have to leave the house to exercise if you don't want to. Pedal on a stationary bicycle; run or jog in place; jump rope, real or imaginary; dance to records; do routine exercises. Keep the body moving—that's the message.

When you quit, most of you will have a hand problem. What do we do with an empty hand? You've been picking up a cigarette, tapping it lightly, putting it back, putting it between your lips, setting it down, picking it up again, puffing away, and forming a repetitive smoking pattern. Over and over and over you have repeated them, day in and day out, for years.

Now you will have to substitute something else to hang onto instead of the customary cigarette. My patients have consistently reported how helpful they have found exercise for blowing off steam and releasing tensions.

Check my suggested exercises (Chapter 14). You can't puff on a cigarette when you're exercising vigorously.

For at least half of you, the side effects of giving up smoking will be tough. But when you make it, I hope you'll all feel like my patient who told me after quitting, "I feel clean. I feel alive. I can run without hesitation. Your work is miraculous."

It may help some, during the first nerve-racking days you have to fight through, if you find someone who will quit smoking when you do. Maybe a family member or a friend, a colleague or a neighbor, will join you. It is often easier for two people to quit together. Misery does love company.

Try to be with nonsmokers as much as possible. Choose people you have fun with and plan to do things that you enjoy.

Do you like to attend concerts, go to dinner, plays, movies, discos, or museums? Ask your nonsmoking pals to go with you. Be good to yourself.

Despite these distractions, the day may come when you will want a cigarette very badly. Strengthen your resolve. Keep your mouth busy with sugarless gum or mints.

Help yourself over this period by changing some of the routines that reinforced your smoking habits for so long. The longer you've smoked, the more firmly entrenched they have become.

Let's review the most common cigarette routines, and try to figure out how to modify them. Coffee and a cigarette, cocktails and a cigarette. You always started a cigarette when you talked on the telephone, after your meals, sometimes first thing in the morning, or the last thing before you turned off the light at night. Before you started a fresh job, you reached for a cigarette, and when you completed a task, you rewarded yourself with a cigarette. These are some of the many usual cigarette-connected actions that my patients have mentioned. One patient said it helped to carry around a small toothbrush and small tube of toothpaste—for brushing after meals instead of reaching for a cigarette. She loved the feeling of knowing she had fresh breath.

If you're alone at mealtime, try to get involved in an exciting book. Having a cocktail or a glass of wine and you're dying for a cigarette? Find a friend—old, new, anyone—who will have some sympathy and talk you through your bad time—especially if your friend is an ex-smoker.

The telephone may pose a particular problem. Hold the phone in your right hand if you've always held a cigarette in it. Use the gum or hard candy or a plastic cigarette you've kept for emergencies. Or try a piece of celery or carrot. Find your own creative ways to deal with your cravings.

One warning. Alert your spouse or lover, your parents, family, and friends that you need them to stand by you, to be tolerant, to accept the irritability that usually accompanies withdrawal. Hopefully this won't last long; it varies from person to person, but you'll need all the understanding you can get. Comfort yourself and them by counting on a longer life, living and loving together. Yes, another real benefit to men who stop smoking is that they may love longer.

"The link between smoking and loss of sexual function is certainly here. We know for instance that peripheral vascular disease (PVD) is more common in smokers." This quote is from Dr. John Rankin of the Wellesley Hospital, Toronto, Canada, in the 1980 newsletter from the Canadian Council on Smoking and Health.

There is evidence that many older men become impotent because of damaged blood vessels serving the genital area. Dr. Rankin noted that PVD is common in the elderly and we don't yet know whether impotence is due to the decreased blood flow to the genital area, but it may be the commonest cause.

He emphasized that PVD is rare in nonsmokers and that most middle-aged men suffering from PVD are smokers. Although the connection has not been proved beyond a shadow of a doubt, why take a chance?

I want to help you. One way is a special alkaline diet I've tailored for smokers trying to kick the habit. I discuss this fully in Chapter 10. It can't take away the craving for tobacco completely, but it cuts down on it.

Prepare yourself by looking at my special diet before you quit. Then be sure to buy whatever foods you need to enable you to follow the menus in Chapter 10. Let this food bolster your resolve by chewing slowly, savoring whatever you are eating. Put your fork down between bites. Chewing keeps your mouth going. As the days go by, your taste buds will come alive again and what you eat will taste so much better.

Finally, let's look forward to a cigarette-free existence, and a healthier life.

5 • Tensions—How to Hurdle

Many mental health professionals consider smoking a form of oral fixation or regression—a throwback to the earliest years of life when, according to psychoanalytic theory, an infant's total gratification is centered around the mouth. Whether or not one completely accepts the Freudian explanation, the fact is that infants do have a well-known propensity for inserting into their mouths any objects they can pick up. Smokers do the same with cigarettes, and ex-smokers demonstrate the same tendency with food. Unlike infants, however, smokers and ex-smokers can be helped to overcome their habits.

Psychoanalytic theory that the continued need for a more infantile form of gratification contributes to habitual smoking takes on credence when one realizes the number of times a smoker has occasion to take a cigarette into his or her mouth. It has been estimated that for the average smoker, this occurs approximately eight times for each cigarette, or one hundred and sixty times for each pack of cigarettes. Since heavy smokers consume more than one pack per day, and do so over a period of several years, it becomes evident that this hand-to-mouth ritual occurs millions of times.

Granted that ex-smokers may continue with their need for oral gratification and attempt to substitute for the cigarettes that previously served this purpose, it does not have to take the form of an increased food intake.

Some persons who want to give up cigarettes but are concerned about putting on excess weight may be helped by behavior modification techniques. For example, for smokers who have developed the habit of having a cigarette with a post-meal cup of coffee, it is important that this association be broken. One simple method of accomplishing this is for the individual to leave the table after a meal and become involved in some other activity.

Hobbyists have a natural outlet; for others, there is always work to be done around the house, a project that should no longer be neglected, or correspondence to be attended to. Not only does involvement in such activities break the coffee-cigarette connection, it also removes the person from the table and from the temptation to continue eating even after nutritional needs have been satisfied.

Paradoxically, those who surrender the post-meal cup of coffee may be faced with another problem. Since caffeine acts as a diuretic, they may experience some degree of fluid retention. This problem is easily resolved by reducing the intake of sodium, which tends to retain fluid in the body, and keeping a supply of low-calorie vegetables on hand. Carrot sticks, celery stalks, and other crunchy items can provide the oral gratification previously obtained from smoking, while contributing to the individual's nutritional well-being. However, if you feel you're a person who can have coffee without reaching for a cigarette, it's OK to continue with the coffee.

Snacking on low-calorie raw vegetables pays an additional bonus. The absence of nicotine, a fairly powerful drug, permits the body to metabolize foods more efficiently. In other words, the same intake of food results in the absorption of more nutrients as well as more calories. Substituting low-calorie items for some of the richer foods a person may have become accustomed to permits a reduction in the amount of calories consumed without creating uncomfortable hunger pangs.

Ex-smokers would also do well to avoid alcohol, at least for the first few weeks of nicotine abstinence. Not only are alcoholic beverages themselves high in calories, they often are linked to the consumption of high-calorie foods—beer with salted pretzels or peanuts, for example. Moreover, too much alcohol may weaken a person's resolve, permitting "just one" cigarette, which may lead to a return to smoking.

Another behavior modification technique is to record all foods eaten during the course of the day, and the circumstances under which the eating occurs—during moments of stress, while watching television, or possibly late at night when one is tired. Obviously, many foods will be consumed during regularly scheduled meals, but people often are surprised when they realize the extent of their food intake simply from snacking.

Many people frequently eat not because they are hungry, but out of a need for some form of gratification which they should be obtaining from other sources. A written record of all foods consumed during the day undercuts the tendency to rationalize that the snacking "really doesn't amount to very much."

A number of my patients have told me they feel compelled to eat when they are tense and anxious. For these people, their weight is actually a barometer of their emotions—that is, as their tensions and anxieties rise, so does their weight; as they learn to relax, their weight goes down.

The National Mental Health Association suggests the following steps a person can take to help relieve stress:

1. Talk it out. When something worries you, don't bottle it up.

2. Escape for a while. When things go wrong, it helps to escape from the painful problem for a while.

3. Work off your anger. Do something constructive with the pent-up energy. Pitch into some physical activity or work it out in tennis or a long walk.

4. Give in occasionally. Even if you're right, it's easier on your system to give in once in a while.

5. Do something for others. If you feel yourself worrying about yourself all the time, try doing something for somebody else.

6. Take one thing at a time. Take a few of the most urgent tasks and pitch into them, one at a time, setting aside all the rest for the time being.

7. Shun the "superman" urge. No one can be perfect in everything.

8. Go easy with your criticism. Each person has his own virtues, his own shortcomings, his own values, his own right to develop as an individual.

9. Give the other fellow a break. When you give the

other fellow a break, you very often make things easier for yourself.

10. Make yourself "available." Instead of shrinking away and withdrawing, it is much healthier, as well as more practical, to continue to make some of the overtures instead of always waiting to be asked.

11. Schedule your recreation. Many people drive themselves so hard that they allow themselves too little time for recreation—an essential for good physical and mental health.

While kicking the smoking habit undoubtedly involves sacrifice, in one sense it should not be considered a sacrifice at all. Those who are motivated to give up their dependence on cigarettes should try to look down the road at the rewards awaiting them—better health, a longer life, and an enhanced sense of well-being. Viewed from this standpoint, ex-smokers are not sacrificing but investing in their futures.

6 • Weighing Too Much

Obesity is an even more common health problem than cigarette smoking. While fifty-four million Americans tempt fate by lighting up, as many as sixty-five million put themselves at risk each time they sit down to a meal.

Twenty years ago, during my training on the Osler Medical Service of the Johns Hopkins Hospital, I was challenged by the myriad problems presented by a 555-pound man who avowedly was committing suicide by eating himself to death. Because of my previous training in physiology (Ph.D. in physiology, with minors in biochemistry and biophysics), I was fascinated by the idea of taking new research laboratory data and applying it clinically to my patient, and I became part of a group of physicians at the Johns Hopkins Hospital who studied this patient for one year.

At the end of that time, we knew what made that patient tick from an endocrinological and metabolic standpoint, had some psychiatric understanding of his problems, and published reports in appropriate medical journals. The patient was treated with the proper medicine, given a specific diet and exercise program, and instructed in behavior modification. I discharged him from the Johns Hopkins Hospital when he weighed 222 pounds.

During that same time, and over the past eighteen years while on the faculty of the Johns Hopkins Medical School, I have continued to try to find out how to get people to lose weight and, more importantly, to keep it off permanently. I coined the term "Yo-Yo Syndrome" for people who repeatedly lose and regain weight. A majority of the patients I now have in my practice in Baltimore come to consult on weight control and endocrinological and metabolic medical problems.

I have seen over one thousand patients with the "Yo-Yo Syndrome," and can tell you that no two people have *exactly* the same basis for their obesity. It is only by working with each individually and treating each of their problems specifically that they can be helped—not all, but a great majority. My method in working with these patients is what I have always advocated—a common sense approach to nutritionally sound eating that becomes a lifetime pattern.

I have incorporated these same principles in my Stop-Smoking, Lose-Weight Diet (Chapter 10).

Based on tables of height, weight, and body build prepared by life insurance actuaries, there is widespread agreement that as many as one-third of the adult population of the United States are overweight; however, there is considerably less agreement as to the cause.

One theory, advanced by Dr. Stanley L. Robbins of the Boston University School of Medicine and Dr. Ramzi S. Cotran of the Harvard Medical School, involves the number of fat cells laid down during three periods of life. In *Pathologic Basis of Disease*, they list these phases as (1) the last three months of pregnancy; (2) the preschool period; and (3) the immediate postpuberty period. According to the theory, an infant born with an excessive number of fat cells, or a child who accumulates excess fat cells during the preschool or immediate postpuberty periods, is destined to be fat, unless they are super-careful calorie counters.

Regardless of a possible constitutional predisposition to obesity, overweight among adults is usually the result of consuming more calories than are expended. If this were merely a cosmetic problem, it would not engender too much concern. But there is evidence that overweight predisposes to a variety of diseases, including high blood pressure, diabetes, heart and blood vessel, and lung disease.

It is a paradox that both starvation and an excess intake of calories are associated with diabetes. In the United States, however, obesity is the main culprit, with about 80 percent of all diabetics significantly overweight. While weight gain may reveal the existence of a disease that had been undetected, loss of weight may change overt diabetes into subclinical, undetected disease.

Excess weight may seriously strain the body. Obese people are more prone to heart and circulation problems, including high blood pressure and stroke, as well as to arthritic complaints and diabetes. They show an increased death rate from cancer, especially that involving the breast, colon, and uterus, and they appear to be more susceptible to infection, especially pneumonia and influenza, and at greater risk for gallbladder and liver disorders. In addition, overweight people tend to suffer more severely from varicose veins, and to be more accident-prone.

In a study conducted by Dr. Ernest J. Drenick, of the

Veterans Administration Wadsworth Hospital Medical Center in Los Angeles, excessive extra weight was shown to increase the risk of early death. Among two hundred men who averaged more than three hundred pounds each, those twenty-five to thirty-four years of age had twelve times the death rate of men of normal weight in the same age bracket. Among those thirty-five to forty-four years old, the death rate was six times higher. Like smoking, obesity can very much be a matter of life and death. However, a recent study by Dr. Reubin Andres of the Johns Hopkins Medical Institution questioned the seriousness of health problems associated with mild and moderate obesity.

Why do people eat? A simple explanation would be that people eat because they are hungry. But while this may be true for most people most of the time, it is not true for all people all of the time.

With obesity this nation's number one nutritional problem as well as its number one chronic illness problem, it is obvious that many individuals consume food well beyond their nutritional requirements.

In addition to eating in order to meet the body's need for energy—that is, for survival—we are influenced by heredity as well as by a host of psychological, social, and cultural factors.

It is apparent that although eating seems to be a simple enough activity—one is hungry, therefore one eats—it involves a complicated process that begins when the brain detects the desire for food, and ends well after the food is ingested.

A person experiences hunger when the body's blood sugar level is low, and usually does not feel hungry when the blood sugar level is high. In a healthy individual, the pancreas releases insulin, which enables the body to use the blood sugar. If there is a relative or absolute deficiency of insulin, as is the case with certain diabetic patients, more blood sugar, instead of being taken into the cells, remains in the blood.

If the theory about the relationship between blood sugar and the sensation of hunger is valid, a person given an injection of insulin, which would lower the blood sugar, would feel hungry—and this is exactly what happens. To summarize: A low blood sugar level stimulates the appetite; a high blood sugar level reduces it.

The portion of the brain that dictates an individual's activity in relation to eating is thought to be the hypothalamus. According to Dr. Timothy J. Teyler, of Harvard University, in his *A Primer of Psychobiology: Brain and Behavior*, two regions of cells within that area appear to be directly concerned with eating behavior. These cells are informed about blood sugar level, stomach contractions, and taste, among other factors.

One of the regions is designated a "stop-eating" center, the other a "start-eating" center. In animal experiments, a hungry rat electrically stimulated in the "stop-eating" area will stop eating even though its hunger has not been assuaged. Conversely, a rat that has eaten its fill will continue to eat when electrically stimulated in the "start-eating" center.

Under normal conditions, the two areas operate reciprocally, so that periods of eating and not eating alternate. The result is called homeostasis—the maintenance of relatively constant conditions within the body.

In other experiments, one or both areas of the hypothalamus, instead of being electrically stimulated, can be surgically removed. A rat in whom the "start-eating" center is missing will not eat even when very hungry and even when offered its most favorite foods. Similarly, a rat without its "stop-eating" center will continue to eat until well beyond its normal weight. This has some relevance to humans, who could very well eat themselves to death.

With many people, putting on weight is an insidious problem. An active eighteen-year-old youngster who is still growing might tolerate a 4,200-calorie diet. Twenty years later, however, the same person may require no more than 2,000 calories daily. Since one pound of fat is deposited for every 3,500 excess calories consumed, the individual who does not alter his diet over the years soon may be faced with a serious weight problem.

Changes in metabolism as one grows older also may lead to a decrease in caloric requirements. Thus, obesity can develop with advancing age even when exercise and food intake remain constant. In my patients I have noticed that this excess weight often is first deposited around the waist in men and in the thighs of women.

In the overwhelming majority of people, weight gain is no mystery. Obesity results when an excess of calories is consumed in relation to the amount expended. A calorie is simply a measure of energy that can be expressed in terms of heat. For example, fat is a high-calorie food; a teaspoonful of butter contains enough calories to raise two-and-one-half pints of water from room temperature to a boil. Proteins and carbohydrates, on the other hand, have less than half the caloric value of fats.

In a small percentage of fat patients—possibly one or two out of a hundred—some endocrine gland disorder may be implicated in cases of obesity. With proper diagnosis and modern treatment methods, a malfunction of the thyroid, pituitary, or other endocrine glands can be remedied, providing the basis for lasting weight reduction.

A small percentage of my fat patients have a low metabolism and an intolerance to certain foods or chemicals.

Very few of these patients (children more often than adults) have an abnormal elevation of a protein called IgE in their blood, and an elevated radioabsorbant serum test (RAST). Elevated IgE and RAST with appropriate signs and symptoms indicates the patient may have an allergy.

I believe that fat patients with a food or chemical intolerance might have a harder time losing weight because of the added stress brought on by the intolerance. Once it is detected through careful history of the patient's medical problems, physical examination, and laboratory tests, the offending agent can be eliminated. In the case of food intolerance, it should simply be eliminated from the diet whenever possible.

There is no clear answer as to *why* people eat beyond their needs. While some undoubtedly tend to overeat when emotionally upset, others find that their appetites are severely depressed when confronting what on the surface, at least, appear to be similar circumstances.

Some individuals eat to excess to compensate for insecurity, anxiety, or loneliness, or as a reaction to emotionally charged experiences, such as illness or the death of a loved one, close friend, or relative. In such cases, the gratification of either conscious or unconscious emotional needs lies at the bottom of the problem.

Some insurance companies and government agencies publish tables that provide a general idea of a person's ideal weight; however, these tables must be interpreted with care. A professional athlete who would be considered overweight according to a table of ideal weights could still be in excellent physical condition, without excess body fat. The weight in these individuals results from unusual muscle development.

The distinction between weight due to fat and that resulting from other causes is important. A person who is gaining weight as a result of fluid retention presents a different medical problem than one with an endocrine gland disorder or a compulsive overeater. Generally, an individual can tell simply by looking in the mirror whether there is a need to take off some weight; flabbiness and a protruding abdomen are fairly reliable signs.

The following rule of thumb may be helpful in determining ideal weight and the amount of calories needed daily:

For a woman, allow 100 pounds for the first five feet of height, and an additional five pounds for every inch over five feet. If the person has a small frame, the total should be decreased by ten percent; a person with a large frame should add ten percent. A woman of average build, five-feet-three-inches in height, should therefore weigh 115 pounds.

For a man, 106 pounds are allowed for the first five feet of height, and six pounds for each additional inch. A five-foot-ten-inch man of average build should weigh about 166 pounds.

To compute the amount of calories needed at complete rest (the basal caloric requirement), simply add a zero to the ideal weight. The total daily caloric requirement for a sedentary person is computed by increasing the basal caloric requirement by one-third; persons who are moderately active should add one-half to obtain their total daily caloric requirement.

Physically active people, such as athletes, who burn up more calories, can double their basal caloric requirement and still maintain their ideal weight.

7 • Group Support and Dieting

There are a number of parallels between the proliferation of smoking cessation programs and those catering to the weight-conscious among us. Dieting, hypnosis, exercise, medication, psychotherapy, acupuncture—even surgery—all have their proponents.

Although a number of voluntary, nonprofit organizations are active in the field, weight control today is in large measure a business venture—in some instances, big business—a not surprising development in a youth-oriented, appearance-conscious society.

Why obesity has become a significant national health problem is readily understandable. The availability of calorie-rich foods, coupled with reduced physical activity as a result of technological advances, provides an ideal setting for the accumulation of fat.

The solution, which is equally understandable, is much easier said than done. Except for a minority of people with metabolic disorders, whether as the result of a glandular deficiency, enzymatic problems such as decreased ATPase activity, or associated with possible food intolerance, the remedy is to reduce caloric intake in relation to caloric expenditures. This can be accomplished through diet, an increase in exercise, or, preferably, a combination of both.

Unfortunately, this formula has led some diet "experts" to conclude that *any* program of weight control that reduces the intake of calories in relation to the amount expended is acceptable. Nothing could be further from the truth. It is a simple matter to design a whole host of diets that would lead to weight loss; unless they were to meet the person's nutritional needs, however, they could have a serious adverse impact on health and, in extreme cases, even result in death. Fad or crash diets have no long-term beneficial effects, and may be harmful.

A good diet is one that not only will lead to loss of weight but, additionally, is nutritionally sound, well balanced, and can be adapted as a pattern to be followed throughout life. It should include education about errors in prior dietary practices, as well as education about sound dietary practices. The patient must learn to eat appropriately, rather than to use food as a means of satisfying nonnutritional needs. And the diet should be based on ordinary foods so that it can be continued with only slight modifications once a desired weight is achieved.

Despite the competitiveness that characterizes so much of business activity in American society, many weight control programs, both commercial and nonprofit, share a number of traits. The most obvious common denominator is the emphasis on group support they provide participants who, notwithstanding an intellectual awareness of what they must do to lose weight, are unable to do so on their own. Behavior modification techniques are another important adjunct of these approaches.

Many of those enrolled in one or another weight control program are sophisticated people, knowledgeable about the need to count calories and the kinds of food to avoid; yet they seem to require the support of a group. Many, who eventually achieve substantial weight loss through an organized program of weight control, acknowledge that they could have followed the same diet on their own. But they had not been able to accomplish by themselves what they were able to do as members of a group.

Among the better known commercial weight control programs are Weight Watchers and the Diet Workshop. Both emphasize group support and behavior modification.

Weight Watchers employs the concept of "food exchanges"—that is, dieters are permitted to substitute one food on a list for any other food on the same list. This provides for greater variety in the diet while maintaining nutritional standards.

Weight Watchers' food exchange lists include fruits; eggs and cheese; bread, cereal, milk, poultry, meat, fish, and legumes; vegetables; and fats. An "optional" group provides for bonus items, such as clam juice, seasoning, condiments, and specialty foods, such as low-calorie jams and jellies. Different menus are prepared for women, men, and youth.

The menus list morning, midday, and evening meals, and dieters are urged never to skip a meal. Although the menus allow for substantial freedom of choice in the selection of foods, some "musts" are set forth. For example, one serving of fruit *must* be taken at the morning meal, vegetables *must* be eaten at the midday and evening meals, and liver *must* be served once a week.

Not required but "strongly recommended" are five fish meals per week; three are "musts," with chicken permitted to be substituted for the one or two fish meals omitted.

The Diet Workshop places a great deal of emphasis on the preparation of popular foods, such as pizza, which usually are high in calories, but using low-calorie recipes. It features six diet programs or "cycles."

"Cycle 1," which furnishes only 750 calories, is designed only for the first week of dieting. Its rationale is that quick weight loss will help provide the motivation for a continuing commitment to dieting. "Cycle 4" is the basic 1,200-calorie diet, and "Cycle 6" covers a four-week maintenance program.

Helen Fleischer, head of the Baltimore Diet Workshop, stresses behavior modification as an aid to dieting. She notes that people who have learned behavior patterns that over the years resulted in overeating and obesity can learn new behavior patterns that will enable them to lose weight and keep it off.

She lists twenty-three behavior options, and suggests that dieters add their own ideas. Some of these behavior modification tips are equally applicable to smokers attempting to give up cigarettes. For example, devoting time to investigating a new hobby or to expanding one's activities can reduce a person's preoccupation with food just as it does with smoking. The behavior modification suggestions follow:

1. I will practice eating as a solitary act.
2. I will eat sitting down only in a proper place.
3. I will stop eating when my body tells me it is satisfied.

4. I will have only low-calorie beverages at between-meal eating segments.
5. I will keep a daily journal of my feelings about dieting.
6. I will use smaller plates.
7. I will leave something on my plate.
8. I will eat slowly and consciously.
9. I will stop and mentally OK food before eating.
10. I will eat only what I've planned in advance.
11. I will put my fork down between bites.
12. I will shop by list only.
13. I will enlist family support.
14. I will plan a weekly menu.
15. I will investigate a new hobby.
16. I will diet 100 percent today.
17. I will include more activity in my life-style.
18. I will tell myself three good things about myself and/or my life each day.
19. I will take time for myself each day.
20. I will eat only off my own plate.
21. I will prepare snacks in advance for coffee breaks.
22. I will prepare my office lunch at home the night before.
23. I will mentally prepare in advance for business luncheons.

Non-commercial organizations devoted to weight control include Overeaters Anonymous (OA), a group consciously patterned after Alcoholics Anonymous (AA), and TOPS, an acronym for Take Off Pounds Sensibly.

OA has adapted AA's twelve steps to recovery to its own use, beginning with: "We admitted we were powerless over food—that our lives had become unmanageable," and ending: "Having had a spiritual awakening as a result of these steps, we tried to carry this message to compulsive overeaters and practice these principles in all our affairs."

TOPS also leans heavily on group support but, in addition, emphasizes competition in weight loss at all levels of operation—chapter, area, state, and national. It scrupulously avoids prescribing diets for its members on the grounds that doing so is a medical responsibility. Continued supervision by a physician during the course of the program is encouraged.

National health organizations, such as the American Diabetic Association (ADA) and the American Heart Association (AHA), have also issued dietary recommendations. The ADA's diet for diabetic patients has been adapted for use in the struggle against obesity. Actually it is not one but several diets, ranging from 1,200 calories—with 125 grams of carbohydrate, 60 grams of protein, and 50 grams of fat—to 3,000 calories—with 300 grams of carbohydrate, 120 grams of protein, and 145 grams of fat. Selection of the appropriate diet is based on the number of pounds that have to be shed for a person to reach an ideal weight.

The ADA diet also employs the food exchange concept. While the proportions of carbohydrate, protein, and fat permitted dieters are controlled, they are permitted to substitute one food on any of six lists for any other food on the same list. The "Bread Exchanges" list, for example, shows that a quarter cup of baked beans can be substituted for one slice of bread.

The AHA's dietary recommendations fall into two categories: avoiding excess weight and reducing the intake of saturated fats and cholesterol. With almost 700,000 deaths from heart attacks each year in the United States, the AHA understandably is concerned about preventive measures.

The AHA diet calls for substituting polyunsaturated fats for saturated fats. The term "saturated" describes the degree to which fats are filled with hydrogen atoms. Fats that are soft or liquid at room temperature, such as corn or safflower oil, are rich in unsaturated fatty acids. Those contained in butter, cheese, and meat, however, which are solid at room temperature, contain mostly saturated fatty acids.

As a physician, I instruct my patients that no matter what diet they use, if they have a strong family history of heart disease or if they themselves have a cholesterol or triglyceride problem, they should substitute polyunsaturated for saturated fats whenever possible.

8 • A Critique of Other Approaches

One of the more drastic efforts to combat morbid (life-threatening) obesity is jejunoileal (intestinal) bypass surgery. The operation permits the foods you eat to bypass most of the small intestines where calories ordinarily are absorbed by the body. Since the calories are not absorbed, weight loss usually results.

Recent evidence suggests that bypass surgery not only is risky, as is all major abdominal surgery, but may have serious adverse side effects that offset any of the procedure's benefits. These include severe diarrhea, vitamin deficiencies, stones in the urinary tract, and accumulation of fat in the liver.

While jejunoileal bypass surgery has resulted in an initial weight loss for many patients, the ultimate success of the operation depends in large part on their eating habits following it. Patients who continue to lose weight after ileal bypass are those who have learned normal eating habits; those who overeat often begin to regain the lost weight, regardless of their initial reaction to the operation.

One study has shown that emotional side effects may accompany the medical ones. Researchers at the University of Kentucky and the University of Wisconsin found striking changes in the relationships between some husbands and wives, including serious marital discord, where one had the operation. For a variety of reasons, the substantial weight loss seemed to upset whatever equilibrium had existed between the spouses.

The medical risks associated with the procedure are sufficient reason to approach it with extreme caution. No one should consider a bypass operation until all nonsurgical efforts at weight loss have been exhausted. Moreover, only patients in whom obesity, itself, is considered a serious threat to health should ever choose this drastic approach to weight loss.

For some people, an alternative to the intestinal bypass operation may be a procedure called gastric (stomach) stapling, which is safer and easier to perform. It is designed to control weight by closing off the greater part of the stomach to create a small pouch that can accept only a limited quantity of food.

The operation involves placing a row of overlapping stainless-steel staples across the upper stomach. A pencil-wide gap is left in the middle of the row to permit food to continue to pass gradually into the body of the stomach. The entire operation takes about an hour, compared with three to five hours for intestinal bypass surgery. Moreover, gastric stapling is a reversible procedure.

Since the operation considerably reduces the capacity for food, patients who consume too much will vomit. In effect, the procedure forces patients to change their eating habits.

As with intestinal bypass surgery, gastric stapling should not be undertaken lightly. One surgeon's criteria in the selection of patients include a weight of at least 100 pounds above normal, and a history of failure on the patient's part to reduce through nonsurgical methods.

The intense desire of some patients to lose weight has led to a number of abuses. Among them is the overprescribing of drugs such as amphetamines, an appetite depressant. The effect of these drugs is temporary, and their use may be habit-forming. I believe the use of medication should be considered only after a thorough history, physical examination, and laboratory tests have shown some imbalance that needs correcting.

Generally, it is preferable to avoid the use of drugs if at all possible. When they are used, proper diet, adequate exercise, behavior modification, and reinforcement of the patient's desire to lose weight are important elements that should not be overlooked. Moreover, appetite suppressant drugs should not be used over an extended period of time, and never without medical supervision. There is no evidence that these drugs contribute significantly to long-term weight reduction.

While a pill may seem rather innocuous, anything that changes the body's chemistry should not be taken lightly or used indiscriminately. Appetite depressants may produce adverse side effects, including insomnia (sleeplessness), nervousness, increased pulse rate, palpitations (heart pounding), and hypertension. It makes no sense to replace one threat to health (obesity) with another (drugs).

Given the urgency with which many people embark on a

program of weight control, sometimes without regard for the consequences, it is not surprising that some potentially harmful regimens have been embraced.

Any program of weight control should be measured in more than the number of pounds lost. Devising a diet that guarantees weight loss is a relatively simple matter. Eating only vegetables and low-calorie liquids will take off pounds, as will a diet of cottage cheese and water, or grapefruit and black coffee, or any one of a number of other imaginative combinations.

But how realistic is it to expect anyone to follow such a diet for any length of time? What happens when we revert to our usual manner of eating? And what is the cost in terms of health in following a diet that not only is low in calories, but in essential vitamins, minerals, and other nutrients as well?

My primary concern with my patients is their health. Although many who come to me want to lose weight for cosmetic reasons—and I don't for a moment minimize the importance of this—my main focus is making them healthier. I do not deal in fad diets or miracle cures.

All weight-reducing diets should meet three criteria; those that do not should be avoided regardless of any claim as to their effectiveness.

First, and most obvious, the diet should provide fewer calories than are expended, so that a loss in weight does in fact occur. Second, it should be nutritionally well-balanced, providing appropriate amounts of protein, carbohydrates, and fat, as well as fiber, vitamins, minerals, and other essential nutrients. And finally, it should be one that patients will be able to follow with only slight modifications once their desired weight is achieved. While a diet of grapefruit and black coffee may meet the first criterion, it certainly doesn't satisfy the other two.

THE PRITIKIN DIET

The Pritikin Diet is based on the theory that an excessive intake of fat and cholesterol is at least partly responsible for a number of degenerative diseases to which humans are subject, including atherosclerosis (hardening of the arteries), hypertension, diabetes, gout, arthritis, and gallstones. Therefore, the diet restricts the daily intake of fat to from five to ten percent of the total, and protein to from ten to fifteen percent. Cholesterol is limited to no more than 100 milligrams a day, and meat and fish to less than 112 grams (slightly less than one-quarter pound) a day. Starches (complex, mostly unrefined carbohydrates) comprise about 80 percent of the total daily intake. Salt is restricted, while coffee, tea, and alcohol are forbidden.

Without arguing about whether an excessive dietary intake of fat and cholesterol is responsible for the diseases listed in the Pritikin program, the main objection to the diet is the difficulty a person would have in adapting it to his or her long-term requirements. Few people will tolerate for any extended period of time a diet that provides the percentages of fat, protein, and carbohydrates called for in the Pritikin Diet. Therefore, even a successful loss of weight is likely to be only a temporary phenomenon as the person gradually reverts to more normal eating habits.

THE SCARSDALE DIET

The Scarsdale Diet calls for 1,000 calories or less per day. It consists of 22.5 percent fat, 43 percent protein, and 34.5 percent carbohydrates—in other words, a high-protein, high-fat, low-carbohydrate diet, when compared to the average American diet.

Although any diet that prescribes a caloric intake of fewer than 1,000 calories a day arouses some concern about its nutritional adequacy, my main objection to the Scarsdale Diet, as to the Pritikin Diet, is that it cannot be adopted as a way of life. Patients who follow diets that produce a loss in weight, only to regain the weight once they resume their customary eating habits, get caught up in my "Yo-Yo Syndrome"—weight loss followed by weight gain followed by weight loss. . . . From a health standpoint, substantial fluctuations in weight may prove more serious than if the patient were to remain at the higher level.

THE STILLMAN DIET

The Stillman or Water Diet is based on the consumption of foods composed mostly of protein. The rationale behind this approach is that more calories are required to burn protein than to burn either carbohydrate or fat.

The diet places no limit on the quantities of food that can be consumed, only on the kinds. Those permitted include lean meats and poultry, lean fish and sea food, eggs, and low-fat cheeses. Foods not permitted include breads and pastries, alcohol, ice cream or sherbet, whole milk or cream, and soft drinks prepared with sugar. Eight glasses of water—in addition to whatever tea, coffee, or diet soda a person drinks—are required each day.

In essence, the Stillman Diet boils down to a protein-and-water diet, with carbohydrates and fats excluded to the extent possible. Obviously, this is not an eating pattern that can easily be—or should be—followed for any length of time.

The diet is monotonous and this, in itself, may cause some people to eat less and therefore lose weight. However, it is deficient in a number of vitamins (A, C, D, and E) and nutrients essential to good health and, because of its restrictions on carbohydrates, may lead to fatigue.

DR. ATKINS' DIET

Dr. Atkins' Diet Revolution is based on the proposition that obesity is related to the inability of a person's body to handle sugar and other carbohydrates; the solution, therefore, is not to cut out calories, but carbohydrates.

After the first week, during which all carbohydrates are eliminated from the diet—but a great deal of fat is consumed—the dieter reaches a second level at which some carbohydrates are permitted. Eventually, the person ascends to "Level Five."

Dr. Atkins emphasizes the state of ketosis—a condition in which fat spills over from the blood into the urine—to which, he says, dieters should aspire since it indicates that fat is being burned. In short, it is claimed, the Diet Revolution enables a person to lose weight by burning fat rather than carbohydrates, and without ever being hungry.

Dr. Atkins' Diet Revolution flies in the face of the American Heart Association's warnings against consumption of large quantities of saturated fats and cholesterol. In addition, in its emphasis on reducing the intake of carbohydrates, it ignores the importance of a diet based on selections from the four food groups—dairy, grain, meat, and fresh fruit and vegetables.

LIQUID PROTEIN DIET

As the name implies, the Liquid Protein Diet consists almost exclusively of protein in liquid form. The obvious criticism of such an approach to weight control is its lack of balance.

A number of nutrients that should be an essential part of everyone's diet simply are not available in liquid protein, even with the use of supplements. In fact, while we know that some foods must contain certain nutrients, at present we do not even know what these nutrients are. What we do know, however, is that they are lacking in the Liquid Protein Diet.

Furthermore, any diet as narrow in scope as this one encourages poor eating habits and cannot be sustained for any extended period of time. While a person may lose some excess poundage on the Liquid Protein Diet because of its limited calorie content, it is not surprising that once the diet has run its course, many people return to their original weight.

Dieters also should bear in mind that the Liquid Protein Diet has been associated with a few deaths due to heart disease.

THE STARVATION DIET

The ultimate in weight reduction is the starvation diet—total fasting. Any such drastic approach to weight loss should be carried out in a hospital under medical supervision. Those who advocate total fasting say it is easily tolerated because patients usually lose their appetites after three or four days; therefore, they feel little discomfort.

The starvation diet may have serious consequences in the absence of medical supervision—problems with the heart, blood pressure, or acute gout. Individuals with a history of heart or liver disease, or gout, should not attempt such a diet.

Although the object of a starvation diet obviously is loss of fat, dieters actually lose a great deal of protein and potassium. A substantial weight reduction is experienced during the first two weeks, but this is caused in large part by a loss of protein and water. Moreover, total fasting does not seem to produce any better or more lasting results than a low-calorie diet. One important problem with this method of weight reduction is that the patient is not trained to handle food in a more reasonable fashion than had previously been the case.

Several years ago I wrote:

> All crash fad diets eliminate some important nutrients your body needs for optimal health. . . . What you want to do is to develop lifelong, sound eating habits, coupled with good exercise. It is impossible to do this on unbalanced diets.

Nothing that has happened since this was written has caused me to change my mind.

9 • Why <u>This</u> Diet?

Many of the people who come to me originally rationalized their past inability or unwillingness to give up cigarettes by maintaining they would gain weight if they stopped smoking. In this fashion, they presented themselves with two unattractive alternatives.

A choice between the lesser of two evils really is no choice at all. But these need not be the alternatives. There *is* a diet that will lead both to weight reduction *and* a decreased desire to smoke.

The Stop-Smoking, Lose-Weight Diet furnishes between 1,300 and 1,400 calories a day. It is well-balanced and nutritious, with none of the gimmicks that result in weight loss at the risk of health. Most importantly, it provides a pattern that can be adapted to your future needs once you have achieved your ideal weight. Since a pound of fat is deposited for every 3,500 excess calories consumed, a diet that provides for 500 calories a day less than the amount expended will lead to a weight loss of a pound a week. But just as the amount of calories people expend varies from person to person, so will the amount of weight loss vary from person to person. Even losing a pound a week means a 20-pound weight loss over twenty weeks, and a 52-pound weight loss over a year.

This diet, in addition to providing all the essential nutrients within a limited number of calories, has an unusual feature. It makes your urine less acidic and therefore more alkaline.

In general, smokers whose urine characteristically is more acidic are expected to smoke more than those whose urine characteristically is more alkaline.

Smokers have a biological craving for nicotine and a consequent need to maintain a given level of the drug in order to keep themselves comfortable. Therefore, someone who has stopped smoking and, as a result, has a precipitous drop in the nicotine level in the blood, is likely to have a strong craving for nicotine. Following a diet that makes the urine more alkaline permits the nicotine to be excreted more slowly, thus lessening the craving.

This approach is based in part on significant studies conducted by Dr. Stanley Schachter and his colleagues at Columbia University, among others.

In *Pharmacological Basis of Therapeutics*, Doctors L. S. Goodman and A. Gilman note that when urine is alkaline, only one-fourth as much nicotine is excreted as when urine is acid. Using these findings and other data, Dr. Schachter estimates that 35 percent of nicotine is excreted when the urine is acid, seven percent when it is neutral, and less than one percent if it is alkaline; the exact proportion will vary with the pH (hydrogen ion concentration) of the urine.

In my practice, I specialize in weight control. When I see people who are also trying to stop smoking, I use a double-barreled approach. In addition to giving a diet based on foods that tend to decrease the acidity of the urine, I prescribe an individually determined amount of baking soda (sodium bicarbonate) to be taken with a glass of water each morning for a week.

Before I do this, however, I obtain a history and perform a physical examination and laboratory tests to make certain there is no heart disease, kidney problems, or high blood pressure. Patients with any of these conditions either should not take baking soda, or the amount prescribed should be modified. If you have any of these problems, you should check with your physician.

If not, after checking with your physician for his approval, you can take one teaspoon of baking soda in an eight-ounce glass of water once a day, or at additional times of overwhelming craving for nicotine. This will further help to alkalinize the urine.

This dietary approach to the dual health risks of obesity and smoking is not a panacea; it cannot and will not help everyone. For example, it will not work in people with metabolic problems; they require medication for their condition in addition to the special diet. Nor will it work for those greatly physically addicted to, or excessively psychologically dependent upon, nicotine; these people may benefit from my stop-smoking injections, a form of treatment discussed in Chapter 12.

The Stop-Smoking, Lose-Weight Diet should help 50 percent of all people who are motivated to stop smoking; of the remaining 50 percent, half should respond to my stop-smoking injections. The remaining 25 percent will not be helped; either they cannot stop smoking, or, if they do, they will gain weight. This may be either because of a metabolic problem that calls for medical intervention, or a psychological problem that may require psychotherapy.

People often ask if increasing fiber in the diet would be useful at this time.

The role of fiber in the diet has been a subject of increasing importance in recent years. While its value has been recognized for some time—years ago it was referred to as "roughage"—today much more is known about its effects on bodily functions.

Until recently, the part played by dietary fiber was largely a neglected subject. Nutritionists understandably pay more attention to the part of the diet that is digestible than to the portion that is not. Most of what we eat is made available for immediate use by the action of digestive enzymes, and this is what usually concerns nutritionists. But the fact that fiber cannot be digested does not mean that it is without dietary value.

What is dietary fiber? Dietary fiber is simply the part of the plant that is not broken down by chemical action during the process of digestion. Some of its components are cellulose, hemicellulose, lignin, and pectin, all resistant to enzymes secreted by the digestive tract. Those who advocate consumption of foods high in fiber—such as bran, whole grains, and many fruits and vegetables—claim its use can prevent a number of diseases, including cancer of the colon, hemorrhoids, appendicitis, varicose veins, and diverticular disease. For some people, a high-fiber diet also may aid in weight control since it requires more chewing and may satisfy hunger more rapidly.

Recognition of the value of dietary fiber is in part an outgrowth of observations by Dr. Denis Burkitt, a British physician who visited my medical office in Baltimore, Maryland, recently. He told me a number of diseases were all but unknown among rural Africans he treated in Uganda. The diseases, however, did occur in Africans who moved to urban areas and began consuming diets low in fiber and high in fat.

Similarly, Dr. Burkitt told me that diseases such as cancer of the colon, diverticular disease, coronary heart disease, and obesity used to be less common among blacks in the United States than among whites. He attributed this to the fact that many blacks lived in rural areas before World War II, and their diets were higher in fiber than those of whites. As the foods they consumed became increasingly like those consumed by whites, the incidence of these diseases in the two groups became virtually the same.

Although some of the claims about the value of a high-fiber diet remain controversial, it does appear to be useful in treating constipation and diverticular (large bowel) disease. This is due to the effect fiber has on the consistency and bulk of stool, and the time it takes to travel through the intestines. Since fiber holds water, stools resulting from high-fiber diets are bulkier and softer, and pass through more easily. Those who champion the use of fiber reason that this action means that bowel tissues are less exposed to poisons and cancer-causing substances produced in the intestines. They also believe it reduces the amount of cholesterol absorbed by the body.

Different plants provide different types of fiber, the amounts also varying from one plant to another. Pectin, the substance that helps convert some fruit juices into jelly, is found in apples, grapes, and some other fruits, while bran is almost entirely cellulose.

The chances are that many people consume more fiber than they realize. Cellulose is used in low-calorie salad dressings, whipped cream toppings, and in some breads, to name only a few products to which it is added. Since it is tasteless and odorless and does not change the color, flavor, or aroma of the food, the additive largely goes unnoticed.

If dietary fiber is as important as many people claim, why isn't it added to more foods? This would be possible to some extent—for example, with breakfast cereals—but in most foods it would not be acceptable to the consumer. To be of any real benefit, fiber would have to be added in amounts that would change the appearance of the food, the way it tastes, and its consistency and texture. Moreover, fiber is sufficiently available in foods such as cereals, fruits, and vegetables, so that its use as an additive is unnecessary in a properly varied diet.

A "properly varied diet" is the key. A person who eats a wide variety of foods, preferably unprocessed, will probably be consuming substantial amounts of fiber. On the other hand, adding fiber to a poor diet will not make it good.

10 • My Stop-Smoking, Lose-Weight Diet

It is a mathematical theorem that the whole equals the sum of its parts. The Stop-Smoking, Lose-Weight Diet, supplemented by exercise and with its emphasis on high-alkaline foods, is greater than the sum of its parts. While each feature of the regimen would be of some value to you who want to break the smoking habit and lose weight at the same time, the total program, when followed by a highly motivated person, increases the possibility of success manyfold.

Once involved in a regularly scheduled exercise program, some of my patients have given up cigarettes simply because they interfered with their enjoyment of physical activity, whether tennis or running or any other. Moreover, exercise itself, since it can be relaxing, may eliminate the desire for cigarettes by otherwise tense individuals. I have had patients tell me that they sleep much better on the days they run, and awaken more refreshed. Some of these same persons had previously sought relaxation, almost always unsuccessfully, at the end of a cigarette.

It is important to remember, however, that exercise complements, but does not substitute for, the Stop-Smoking, Lose-Weight Diet. The diet provides nutritional, well-balanced meals totaling between 1,300 and 1,400 calories a day, with an emphasis on high-alkaline foods. These include fruits, vegetables, milk, and nuts, such as almonds, chestnuts, and coconut. To repeat the rationale for such a diet: A high-alkaline diet permits a slow, steady release of nicotine from the system, rather than a precipitous drop that only triggers the craving for additional nicotine and, thus, leads to a resumption of smoking.

In general, green salads featuring lettuce, tomatoes, celery, and cucumbers are both low in calories and high in alkaline content. By the same token, a dessert of cooked dried apricots, which is alkaline, is lower in calories than a piece of chocolate cake, which is acidic. The same is true of other fruits and melons—apples, cherries, cantaloupes, peaches, and pears, to name a few.

You dieters need not stick exclusively to high-alkaline foods. This is neither desirable nor necessary. A sound regimen must be based on the selection of a variety of foods from each of the four food groups. But a serving of pineapple can easily be substituted for a portion of high-calorie, acidic pastry.

The basic 1,300 to 1,400 calorie Stop-Smoking, Lose-Weight Diet consists of 46 grams of fat, 78 grams of protein, and 156 grams of carbohydrate, the majority complex carbohydrates. The diet is relatively high in complex carbohydrate since these foods generally produce an alkaline ash, and relatively low in protein because such foods generally produce an acidic ash. You need to follow the diet for a minimum of twenty-eight days in order to allow the nicotine to leave your system gradually, thus lessening craving. If more weight loss is desired, you can continue with this or any other well-balanced reducing diet.

Following are some of the main features of my Stop-Smoking, Lose-Weight Diet:

- Milk, which provides about one-half the complete and essential amino acids, also furnishes needed calcium, vitamin D, and vitamin A.

- Fruits (except for prunes, plums, and cranberries) and vegetables (except for corn, dried peas, beans, and lentils) provide sodium, potassium, and magnesium. Vegetable salads should include several varieties of lettuce to increase taste sensations, and some chopped greens such as spinach. Cauliflower, tomato, broccoli, and cucumbers provide color, the sensation of chewing, and sound.

- Drink four to five glasses of water each day in addition to the liquids included at meals. In all, you should have at least eight glasses of liquid a day. If you use coffee, the decaffeinated type is preferred.

- Orange juice, grapefruit, and/or cantaloupe should be part of your daily diet because of their potassium and vitamin C content.

- Low-calorie lemonade is recommended. It helps provide the fluids needed and gives an additional alkaline reaction. You can drink lemonade at any time during the day. Try the following recipe:

    1 tablespoon fresh or reconstituted lemon juice
    artificial sweetener to taste
    8 ounces cold water
    add lemon wedge or mint sprig for color, if desired

- Try adding tomato or V-8 juice at noon, although either one can also be used in the evening. They increase the alkaline reaction desired, and can be served hot with a wedge of lemon or lime.

- Most noon meals assume that lunch will be brought to work. This lessens the temptation to overbuy in fast-food or other restaurants. The sight and odor of food plus the presence of other smokers might present problems, especially for the person just starting on the diet.

- Meats, fish, poultry, and cheeses yield an acidic ash; therefore, limit your consumption of these. If you increase your intake of such foods, you alter the pH levels significantly.

- The 1,300 to 1,400 calories provided are slightly more than the basic 1,200-calorie weight reduction diet in order to allow you greater variety. Women are encouraged to follow the diet as presented; men who are not overweight may add an additional ounce of meat and one fruit each day. These changes would add about 110 calories. However, overweight men should follow the prescribed diet.

Menu suggestions for a fourteen-day period follow. Items marked with an asterisk(*) have an alkaline reaction. You do not have to eat everything on the menu, but try to eat all items marked with an asterisk.

DAY 1

Breakfast

½ cantaloupe*
1 boiled egg
1 white toast
1 cup skim milk*
coffee or tea

Lunch

½ cup tomato/V-8 juice*
2 ounces cheddar cheese
large, mixed raw vegetable salad*
low-calorie dressing
4 saltines
1 cup low-calorie lemonade*

Dinner

3 ounces pot roast
½ cup mashed potato*
1 cup broccoli*
large, mixed raw vegetable salad*
low-calorie dressing
1 teaspoon margarine
6 dried apricots*
beverage

Snack

1 cup skim milk*

DAY 2

Breakfast

½ cup orange juice*
¾ cup corn flakes
1 cup skim milk*
coffee or tea

Lunch

½ cup tomato/V-8 juice*
½ cup cottage cheese
large, mixed raw vegetable salad*
low-calorie dressing
3 Rye Krisp
low-calorie lemonade*

Dinner

3 ounces baked chicken
½ cup rice
1 cup beets*
large, mixed raw vegetable salad*
low-calorie dressing
1 teaspoon margarine
2 figs*
beverage

Snack

1 cup skim milk*

DAY 3

Breakfast

½ grapefruit*
1 egg, scrambled, without fat
1 slice white toast
1 cup skim milk*
beverage

Lunch

½ cup tomato/V-8 juice*
large, mixed raw vegetable salad*
1 ounce cheddar cheese, sliced
1 ounce ham, sliced
2 bread sticks
3 slices pineapple, without sugar*
beverage

Dinner

3 ounces roast veal
½ cup oven-browned potato*
1 cup Swiss chard or spinach*
large, mixed raw vegetable salad*
low-calorie dressing
1 teaspoon margarine
½ cup canned cherries*

Snack

1 cup skim milk*

DAY 4

Breakfast

½ banana
¾ cup corn flakes
1 cup skim milk*
beverage

Lunch

½ cup tomato/V-8 juice*
½ cup tuna fish
1 large tomato, sliced*
cucumber slices*
1 orange*
beverage

Dinner

3 ounces baked fish, with lemon
½ cup carrots*
½ cup lima beans*
large, mixed raw vegetable salad*
low-calorie dressing
1 teaspoon margarine
½ broiled grapefruit*

Snack

1 cup skim milk*

DAY 5

Breakfast

1 cup applesauce*
½ cup Farina cereal
1 tablespoon molasses*
1 cup skim milk*
beverage

Lunch

½ cup tomato/V-8 juice*
1 egg, made into salad
½ teaspoon mayonnaise
celery, carrot sticks*
large, mixed raw vegetable salad*
1 cup low-calorie lemonade*
3 tablespoons raisins*
beverage

Dinner

3 ounces lean fresh ham
1 cup sauerkraut*
½ cup boiled potato*
large, mixed raw vegetable salad*
low-calorie dressing
1 teaspoon margarine
1 fresh pear*
beverage

Snack

1 cup skim milk*

DAY 6

Breakfast

    ½ cup canned or stewed apricots, without sugar*
    1 egg, poached
    1 slice rye toast
    1 cup skim milk*
    beverage

Lunch

    ½ cup tomato/V-8 juice*
    2 ounces cold roast beef
    large, mixed raw vegetable salad*
    low-calorie dressing
    1 cup low-calorie lemonade*
    1 raw apple*
    beverage

Dinner

    3 ounces meat loaf
    1 cup green beans*
    1 small baked potato*
    large, mixed raw vegetable salad*
    low-calorie dressing
    1 teaspoon margarine
    1 cup strawberries, without sugar*
    beverage

Snack

    1 cup skim milk*

DAY 7

Breakfast

½ cup orange juice*
¾ cup high-vitamin/mineral cereal
1 cup skim milk*
beverage

Lunch

½ cup tomato/V-8 juice*
5 medium shrimp, hot sauce to taste
large, mixed raw vegetable salad*
3 Rye Krisp
1 cup low-calorie lemonade*
½ cup seedless grapes*
beverage

Dinner

3 ounces lean corned beef
1 cup steamed cabbage*
½ cup parsley carrots*
large, mixed raw vegetable salad*
low-calorie dressing
1 teaspoon margarine
1 large tangerine*
beverage

Snack

1 cup skim milk*

DAY 8

Breakfast

½ cup grapefruit juice*
1 egg, scrambled, no fat
½ English muffin
1 cup skim milk*
beverage

Lunch

½ cup tomato/V-8 juice*
1 ounce cold cut
1 ounce sliced cheese
large, mixed raw vegetable salad*
low-calorie dressing
1 cup low-calorie lemonade*
½ cantaloupe*
beverage

Dinner

3 ounces lean broiled steak
1 small baked potato*
1 cup asparagus*
large, mixed raw vegetable salad*
low-calorie dressing
1 teaspoon margarine
1 cup blackberries, fresh/frozen*
beverage

Snack

1 cup skim milk*

DAY 9

Breakfast

½ cup blueberries*
¾ cup corn flakes
1 cup skim milk*
beverage

Lunch

½ cup tomato/V-8 juice*
chef's salad with:
  1 hard-boiled egg
  1 ounce sliced ham
  low-calorie dressing
5 Triscuits
1 fresh orange*
beverage

Dinner

Pepper steak:
  3 ounces thinly sliced beef
  1 green pepper, chopped
  1 tablespoon corn starch
  ½ cup steamed rice
1 cup carrots*
large, mixed raw vegetable salad*
low-calorie dressing
1 teaspoon margarine
1 baked apple*
beverage

Snack

1 cup skim milk*

DAY 10

Breakfast

½ cup orange juice*
1 egg, boiled
1 slice toast
1 cup skim milk*
beverage

Lunch

½ cup tomato/V-8 juice*
1 broiled hot dog
½ roll, toasted
large, mixed raw vegetable salad*
low-calorie dressing
1 cup low-calorie lemonade*
2 fresh plums
beverage

Dinner

3 ounces broiled chicken
¼ cup fresh mushrooms
1 cup greens—spinach, kale, Swiss chard*
¼ cup sweet potato*
large, mixed raw vegetable salad*
low-calorie dressing
1 teaspoon margarine
1 cup watermelon*
beverage

Snack

1 cup skim milk*

DAY 11

Breakfast

½ cup grapefruit juice*
2 shredded wheat biscuits
1 cup skim milk*
beverage

Lunch

½ cup tomato/V-8 juice*
Sandwich:
   3 strips bacon
   1 tomato, sliced*
   lettuce, ½ teaspoon mayonnaise
   1 slice bread
large, mixed raw vegetable salad*
low-calorie dressing
1 cup raspberries, fresh/frozen*
beverage

Dinner

3 ounces broiled veal chop
1 cup broccoli*
½ cup mashed potato*
large, mixed raw vegetable salad*
low-calorie dressing
1 teaspoon margarine
½ cup canned or stewed apricots*
beverage

Snack

1 cup skim milk*

DAY 12

Breakfast

½ cup mixed fruit juice*
1 egg, boiled
1 cup skim milk*
beverage

Lunch

½ cup tomato/V-8 juice*
2 ounces fast-food hamburger
½ roll
large, mixed raw vegetable salad*
low-calorie dressing
½ grapefruit*
beverage

Dinner

3 ounces roast turkey
low-calorie cranberry sauce
1 cup asparagus*
½ cup boiled potato*
large, mixed raw vegetable salad*
low-calorie dressing
1 teaspoon margarine
1 cup orange/grapefruit sections*
beverage

Snack

1 cup skim milk*

DAY 13

Breakfast

½ cup orange juice*
¾ cup cereal
1 cup skim milk*
beverage

Lunch

½ cup tomato/V-8 juice*
½ cup water-packed tuna, stuffed into large tomato
large, mixed raw vegetable salad*
1 cup skim milk*
¼ fresh cantaloupe, with lemon wedge*
beverage

Dinner

1 medium chicken breast (baked), prepared with tomato sauce
½ cup rice
½ cup broccoli, with lemon wedge*
½ cup carrots, with chopped parsley*
large, mixed raw vegetable salad*
1 teaspoon margarine
½ fresh grapefruit*
beverage

Snack

1 cup skim milk*
2 unsweetened peach halves
Blend into a fruit/milk drink

DAY 14

Breakfast

    2 pineapple slices, no added sugar*
    1 boiled egg
    1 white toast
    1 cup skim milk*
    beverage

Lunch

    ½ cup tomato/V-8 juice*
    ½ cup cottage cheese
    large, mixed raw vegetable salad*
    low-calorie dressing
    3 Rye Krisp
    low-calorie lemonade*

Dinner

    3 ounces baked chicken
    ½ cup mashed potato*
    1 cup broccoli*
    large, mixed raw vegetable salad*
    low-calorie dressing
    1 teaspoon margarine
    4 dried apricots*
    beverage

Snack

    1 cup skim milk*

After you have been on my Stop-Smoking, Lose-Weight Diet for fourteen days, repeat it for an additional fourteen days. After twenty-eight days on the diet, a number of you will have stopped smoking and lost weight.

If some of these meals don't appeal to you, you can make your own using this guide:

Breakfast

½ cup orange juice or ½ fresh grapefruit
¾ cup high-vitamin/mineral cereal
1 cup skim milk
coffee, tea, decaffeinated coffee

Some of you may not wish to drink all of the skim milk at breakfast, or you may not enjoy drinking black coffee. The morning milk allowance may be used in coffee or tea during the day.

Fruit Choices

½ cup orange juice or ½ cup grapefruit juice
1 fresh peach, pear, apple, orange, apricot, or tangerine
¼ fresh cantaloupe or honeydew melon
2 canned (sugar-free) peach halves, pear halves, apricot halves, or pineapple slices
½ cup unsweetened applesauce, grapefruit sections, or orange sections

Vegetable Salad

(For lunch or dinner, should include any or all)
lettuce, romaine, endive, Chinese cabbage, radish, watercress
fresh greens, such as kale, spinach, beet greens
bean sprouts, alfalfa sprouts
green pepper chunks
tomato wedges
sliced mushrooms
raw broccoli
cauliflower buds
cucumbers

Lunch

Choose one of the following protein products (may be hot or cold):
½ cup low-fat cottage cheese
½ cup water-packed tuna or salmon
2 slices lean roast beef or roast veal
2 slices roast turkey or chicken, without skin
1 egg—boiled, poached, hard-boiled, soft-boiled
1 slice low-fat cheese food
5 small boiled shrimp

Choose one of the following vegetables (may be hot or cold). One cup served without butter or margarine:

asparagus	cauliflower	beans—string or wax
beets	celery	yellow squash

broccoli	cucumbers	zucchini squash
carrots	greens	sauerkraut
tomatoes	tomato juice	V-8 juice
turnips		
okra	rutabaga	

Include at least one cup of vegetable salad.

Salad dressing should be a good low-calorie product, with no more than one tablespoon used with each serving.

1 cup of skim milk or 1 cup plain low-fat yogurt
One choice from any of the fruits listed

If yogurt is chosen in place of milk, fresh or unsweetened canned fruit can be added to it for dessert.

Beverage:
diet soda, coffee, tea, low-calorie lemonade

Dinner

Choose one of the following protein products; meat products may be baked, broiled, roasted, or steamed.

All visible fat should be removed prior to cooking, and skin should be removed from poultry products prior to cooking.

3 ounces of lean roast beef, corned beef, ground round steak, tenderloin, or rib roast

3 ounces veal—leg, loin, shank, cutlets
3 ounces poultry—chicken, turkey, cornish hen, pheasant
3 ounces pork (limited to no more than once a week)—loin, shoulder arm roast, lean chops, ground ham, or center ham slices

Vegetables should be selected from the luncheon list; one full cup permitted.

Salad is the same as the luncheon choice; one full cup permitted.

One teaspoon of margarine is permitted, but may be omitted.

For starch, choose one of the following foods in the amount shown:

1/2 cup mashed potato
1 small baked potato
1/4 cup sweet potato
1/2 cup green peas
1/2 cup lima beans
1 slice white, rye, pumpernickel, or whole wheat bread
1/2 hamburger bun
1/2 plain or onion bagel
1 small dinner roll
1/2 cup rice
1 small boiled potato
1/2 cup noodles

Select fruit from those previously listed.

P.M. Snack

1 cup skim milk or 1 cup plain yogurt

Some individuals seem to be able to stop smoking and not gain weight. To these people, let me emphasize the necessity of following the basic diet plan. Since meat, fish, eggs, and poultry products produce an acid ash, adhering to the diet will insure the desired alkaline ash reaction. If weight is not a problem, fruits, juices, vegetables, hard candy, milk, yogurt, bread or rolls with margarine may be eaten as desired. They will increase the total caloric level without changing the needed alkaline reaction.

Some smokers who have tried to quit resumed the habit because they could not tolerate the withdrawal pangs as the nicotine left their system. The Stop-Smoking, Lose-Weight Diet, with its emphasis on foods with a high-alkaline content, slows down the loss of nicotine and thus helps minimize these symptoms. Those who feel ill-at-ease or short-tempered at the outset of the smoking cessation program should try to bear in mind that these are temporary discomforts, a roadblock to be overcome on the way to a longer, healthier life.

In addition to adopting the Stop-Smoking, Lose-Weight Diet, ex-smokers can minimize withdrawal symptoms by following some common sense health habits—getting sufficient rest; increasing their intake of fluids such as water (which increases circulation and stimulates digestion), milk (which helps soothe nerves and combats fatigue), and citrus and tomato juices (which provide energy); giving themselves some pleasurable activity each day, including sex; and following a regular exercise program as discussed in Chapter 14.

11 • A French Connection

I expect the majority of you will stop smoking on your own, if indeed you have not already done so. For those who can't, here's the way I help people who come to me, and how it came about.

Like so many other medical procedures discovered by accident, the origin of the stop-smoking shots was a serendipitous experience of a French physician, Dr. Michel Bicheron. The element of chance was further compounded by the fact that I learned of the technique through a patient under my care, rather than through the usual sources of medical information—that is, a conference or professional journal.

My patient was a forty-two-year-old man who had been referred for a program of diet and weight control following his recovery from a massive heart attack. He had a history of smoking two to three packs of cigarettes a day over a period of fifteen years, and his symptoms bore this out. They included morning cough and an almost constant wheeze, and although he was twenty-five pounds overweight, he complained of a decreased taste for food.

On physical examination, the patient had moderately high blood pressure, an expanded chest with decreased breath sounds, and was pre-emphysematous. After completion of the patient's medical history, physical examination, urinalysis, pulmonary function tests, and an electrocardiogram, his ideal weight was determined, and a diet prescribed.

While he seemed resigned to the need to lose weight and indicated a readiness to adhere to the prescribed diet, he failed in several attempts to stop smoking even though he was well aware of the damaging effects of cigarettes on his heart. We both knew that the combination of risk factors—the previous heart attack and his moderately high blood pressure and obesity—was sufficiently threatening without the additional burden of a two- to three-pack-a-day habit.

In view of the seriousness of the situation, and in an effort to help him stop smoking or at least get him to curtail the habit, I began exploring the more popular stop-smoking methods in use. My investigation soon revealed that, despite the proliferation of smoking cessation programs in recent years, conventional approaches to the problem were not very successful.

According to the National Cancer Institute, 90 percent of the fifty-four million Americans who smoke would like to break the habit but are unable to do so. Furthermore, only two percent of those who want to quit are sufficiently motivated even to enroll in a formal program.

Addiction to smoking is a multifaceted problem based

on complex physiological and psychological mechanisms. As previously noted, nicotine can act as a stimulant, depressant, or tranquilizer, depending on the dosage. The smoker who is really hooked unconsciously consumes cigarettes at a rate that provides the level of nicotine required by the brain to produce the desired effect.

Ignoring reason and my warnings and efforts at persuasion, the patient continued to smoke. But although he was unable to take positive action in what, for him, was a matter of life and death, it was information he dropped almost casually that led me on a trip to Paris and the development of the stop-smoking shots.

During one of his office visits, the patient mentioned that he had heard of an approach developed by a French physician that enabled many people to stop smoking in a single day. My initial reaction was one of profound skepticism. In the first place, it seemed too good to be true, and I was tempted to place this "cure" in the same category as the use of copper bracelets for the treatment of arthritis. The treatment may be profitable for those who sell copper bracelets; it has no proven beneficial effect on patients.

Secondly, I had neither read nor heard anything about such a procedure in any of the medical journals and research papers that I study continually.

And finally, I had the distinct impression that the patient was grasping at straws, looking for an easy way out of a dilemma that I felt could be resolved only by willpower and a determination to stop smoking.

These early doubts were reinforced when my efforts to obtain additional information about the procedure drew a blank. None of those with whom I spoke at the National Cancer Institute, the American Cancer Society, or the American Medical Association, nor my colleagues at the

Johns Hopkins School of Medicine, had ever heard of the method or of Dr. Bicheron.

Having gone this far, however, I decided to pursue the subject a little further; the potential for a simple, effective cure for smoking was too appealing to be dismissed out of hand. I decided to follow the lead to its source. The next step was a transatlantic telephone conversation through an interpreter with Dr. Bicheron in Paris.

Dr. Bicheron was gracious and cooperative over the phone. He informed me he had used the stop-smoking procedure on more than 4,000 patients over a period of four years. In addition, he had trained other physicians, who subsequently introduced the technique in other European cities, including Nice, Rome, and Brussels. In all, some 12,000 people were said to have been treated, 85 percent of them successfully.

"Success" in this instance was defined by him as cessation from smoking for a period of up to one month, the extent of Dr. Bicheron's follow-up. Encouraged by this conversation, but with my doubts only slightly allayed, I decided to pursue the subject on a more personal level and arranged to meet with Dr. Bicheron in Paris.

In March 1979 I went to Paris. The following morning, I arrived at the Centre Medical Miromesnil, a large clinic with a staff of about thirty doctors, where I met Dr. Michel Bicheron, the director of the mesotherapy unit.

I can best describe Dr. Bicheron as "typically French"—a tall, slim, balding, very distinguished-looking gentleman in a white lab coat, a stethoscope around his neck, and a monocle in one eye. Aside from his medical exploits, Dr. Bicheron is best known in Paris for having established the first "expedition by horseback" for tourists—an opportunity for travelers with a flare for the unusual to tour France in the saddle. Since Dr. Bicheron speaks English about as well as I speak French—which is not well at all—our conversations were carried on through an interpreter.

I spent a week at the clinic. I learned that Dr. Bicheron's stop-smoking technique developed from a fortuitous set of circumstances. On various occasions, he had noticed a wire hung from an ear of several of his patients. When he inquired about the reason for the wire, he was told it was a form of acupuncture to get people to stop smoking. He said the method had a success rate of about 30 percent, but only worked in motivated people.

There were other coincidences as well. A specialist in the treatment of arthritis, Dr. Bicheron had been injecting into the affected joints of his patients a mixture of vitamins, minerals, and sodium bicarbonate in a procaine base—standard treatment for arthritis by some Parisian physicians for more than forty years according to the doctor. Over a period of time, a number of his arthritic patients had told him that one of the side effects of the treatment was a decreased desire to smoke.

His curiosity piqued, Dr. Bicheron began investigating other methods being used to help people stop smoking. The search led eventually to one of his colleagues at the clinic, an acupuncturist, who claimed to achieve a modicum of success (30 percent) by inserting needles at four acupuncture points—one in the outer aspect of each ear, and one in the outer aspect of each side of the nose.

If his mixture and the acupuncturist's needles both produced favorable results when used separately, Dr. Bicheron reasoned, might they not act synergistically—that is, each enhance the effect of the other—if used together? Putting theory into practice, he injected his mixture into the four acupuncture points instead of into the joints; and although his patients had not been informed of the purpose of the injections—and thus could not have been responding only to a placebo effect—he said that 85 percent reported during subsequent interviews that they had lost their desire to smoke. Their arthritis, however, had not been alleviated with the antismoking shots.

According to Dr. Bicheron, of those treated successfully, ten percent regressed and required a booster shot before their addiction to cigarettes ended. Fifteen percent of the total remained dependent on tobacco, although he believed that the physical craving for nicotine had been eased. Side effects in all cases were negligible. Incidentally, Dr. Bicheron told me that the procedure is covered in France by National Health Insurance.

During my week at the clinic, I learned that many patients referred to Dr. Bicheron suffer from poor circulation related, in part, to their smoking. I had the opportunity to visit and speak with Dr. Regis A. Thierree, professor of radiology at L'Hopital Necker, who was conducting a study of blood flow in these patients by means of thermography, a technique for recording variations in body temperature. His findings showed quite clearly that circulation to various parts of the body increased in patients who stopped smoking.

In May 1979, after I had returned to the United States, I reciprocated Dr. Bicheron's hospitality by inviting him to meet with a small group of physicians at the Johns Hopkins Hospital in Baltimore. While he was received there cordially, the physicians posed a number of difficult questions, many of which I had raised myself.

Did Dr. Bicheron do a controlled study? Had he done a double-blind study (one in which neither patient nor physician knows who receives the active medication, and who receives a placebo)? What is the mechanism of action of the mixture? Why does it work?

In response, Dr. Bicheron could say only that he had not done any studies, controlled or otherwise; that his assessment of the value of the procedure was based on anecdotal information; and that, in essence, all he could conclude about his stop-smoking technique was that it works.

12 • Stop Smoking in Only One Day?

Stop smoking in only one day? Many of you might be tempted to respond with the name of a popular television program on which I recently appeared—"That's Incredible." While it may sound incredible, however, it may nonetheless be true.

Medical procedures generally do not come into being fully developed, like Athena who sprang full-grown from the brain of Zeus. Rather, they are refined painstakingly, often over extended periods of time, each physician building on the efforts of those who preceded him.

This philosophy certainly applies to the procedure I call the stop-smoking shots. While Dr. Bicheron was the first to recognize its value, the method I use in my private practice in Baltimore is substantially different from his. In effect, I have improved on his original and creative discoveries.

My antismoking treatment is not so much a discovery as

a synthesis. Just as any researcher selects and combines and recombines in various ways the components of a treatment, I have borrowed from a variety of sources to improve and refine my antismoking treatment, and have blended them together into a form of treatment that appears to work for many people.

In addition to borrowing from Dr. Bicheron's pioneering method, I have incorporated appropriate portions of allergy methods, called Serial Dilution Antigen Endpoint Titration (SDAET), and provocative testing for tobacco and tobacco smoke. In addition, I utilized some research findings of Dr. Stanley Schachter and his colleagues (see Chapter 9) and strengthened these findings by my own experience in the fields of endocrinologic and metabolic disorders, allergy, and nutrition.

The modifications to Dr. Bicheron's technique that I have introduced encompass three areas: (1) urine alkalinization; (2) some instruction in behavior modification; and (3) provocative intradermal testing for tobacco and tobacco smoke.

The rationale for urine alkalinization is based on an assumption that smokers have a biological craving for nicotine, and a consequent need to maintain a given level of the drug in the blood in order to feel comfortable. Furthermore, studies have indicated that the level of nicotine in a smoker's system is decreased by such factors as stress, alcohol, and the consumption of acidic foods. Decreasing the acidity in a smoker's system permits a slow, steady release of nicotine from the urine, rather than a precipitous drop, thus decreasing the craving for the drug.

A study similar to one by Dr. Schachter and his colleagues at Columbia University was performed by James Fix, Ph.D., at the University of Nebraska. The majority of a group of students who were given sodium bicarbonate, a highly alkaline compound, reported a decreased desire to smoke.

Fortunately for proponents of this theory, sodium bicarbonate is not an absolutely essential part of the treatment. Highly alkaline foods, such as vegetables, which are both nutritious and low in calories, can be used instead. The Stop-Smoking, Lose-Weight Diet you can follow for yourself was discussed in more detail in Chapter 10.

In addition to prescribing an appropriate diet for each of my patients, based on such considerations as their overall nutritional needs, food likes and dislikes, and need to lose weight, I may instruct them to take an individually determined amount of baking soda mixed with water each morning for a period of one week. This more quickly alkalinizes the patient's urine and permits the slow, steady release of nicotine.

My refinement of Dr. Bicheron's technique also includes behavior modification. While Dr. Bicheron's method takes into account the physical basis of a smoker's addiction, it does not deal with the psychological aspects. For starters, there is a sign in the outer hall outside my office requesting patients to deposit all cigarettes there.

I also review with them the circumstances under which they are most likely to reach for a cigarette—for example, while speaking on the telephone—and suggest alternate forms of behavior. For those who smoke out of a need for oral gratification, I recommend eating crunchy vegetables such as celery, carrots, or lettuce, instead. Some of my patients have informed me that sugarless gum, candy mints, cinnamon sticks, and cloves also are satisfactory alternatives to puffing on a cigarette.

My third modification of Dr. Bicheron's technique is provocative intradermal testing for tobacco and tobacco smoke. This method involves giving the patient a series of intradermal injections of tobacco and tobacco smoke extract in varying concentrations. If symptoms are provoked, they are then reversed by administering a treatment dose of the extract. The treatment dose is the highest concentration the patient can tolerate that does not evoke a systemic reaction. Although I use intradermal injections of tobacco and tobacco smoke extract to provoke symptoms, I use shots in the arm or drops under the tongue for the treatment itself.

As is my practice with all my patients, the complete protocol for treating those who come to me because they want to stop smoking begins with the taking of an in-depth medical history and a physical examination. Urinalysis, blood tests, an electrocardiogram, and a pulmonary (lung) function test indicate the extent of the damage, if any, and show the degree to which the damage is reversible. Provocative testing for tobacco and tobacco smoke and treatment follow.

The core of the treatment protocol—the injection of a mixture of vitamin B_1 (thiamin) and procaine in the four acupuncture points, plus an additional shot in the arm—concludes the office procedure. The patient is then given instructions detailing the amount of sodium bicarbonate to be taken daily during the ensuing week, and advised of the need to drink a quart of water each day during this period to help flush the nicotine from the tissues. The session ends with instruction about behavior modification.

13 • Proof of the Pudding

I have treated over 1,000 patients in the past twenty months, ranging in age from teen-agers to senior citizens, who had smoked cigarettes for as long as fifty-eight years. The results have been promising, both in terms of weight loss and smoking cessation.

One question I considered at the very outset, when the Stop-Smoking, Lose-Weight Diet was still being formulated, was whether it was advisable to treat obesity and smoking addiction at the same time. Initially, I was concerned that efforts to treat one condition might interfere with efforts to treat the other. I learned that the reverse was in fact the case—that in regard to smoking cessation and weight control, successful treatment of one reinforced the other.

For example, some patients rationalize that giving up smoking inevitably results in a gain in weight. This, in turn, leads to their further rationalization that since overweight itself is a threat to health, they might as well continue to smoke.

A study by the former Department of Health, Education, and Welfare (HEW) noted that fear of gaining weight discourages many people from giving up cigarettes. In response to an HEW questionnaire, 50 percent of the men and 60 percent of the women surveyed expressed this belief. Surprisingly, more nonsmokers (57 percent) than smokers (53 percent) held this opinion.

Combating obesity and smoking at the same time served to cut through this rationalization. Rather than offering a Hobson's choice between one or the other, this dual approach enabled one to reinforce the other. The validity of this line of reasoning is reflected in the results.

In one series of two hundred and seven patients treated, one hundred and five stopped smoking and have continued to abstain from cigarettes for at least three months. After that period, all indications were that the nicotine had been flushed from their systems, and that their physical craving for cigarettes was gone. Moreover, during the course of treatment they averaged a weight loss of 3.4 pounds per month.

It cannot be overemphasized that those who were successful in kicking the smoking habit were highly motivated people. But while this undoubtedly was the single most important reason for their success, it would not have been sufficient by itself. In fact, many who were successful with the Stop-Smoking, Lose-Weight Diet had made several prior unsuccessful attempts to stop smoking.

In addition to the diet which, as described in Chapter 10, is designed to decrease the acidity of the system, behavior modification techniques played an important role.

Here, too, the two goals—weight control and smoking cessation—complemented each other.

A number of patients reported being helped by behavior modification techniques such as taking up a new hobby, putting more activity into their life-styles, telling themsleves a good thing about themselves and/or their lives each day, and finally by taking time for themselves each day. An interesting idea suggested by Francis Rackemann, a columnist for the *Baltimore Evening Sun*, which has helped a number of patients is holding a piece of a drinking straw in the mouth and sucking on it.

In addition, some of my patients used external support available in the form of a "buddy system," an arrangement that permitted a person who felt the need to smoke to phone and obtain emotional reinforcement from someone who had successfully weathered similar situations. This had a great deal of meaning for some patients.

For the one hundred and two patients for whom diet alone, or behavior modification alone, or diet plus behavior modification did not prove successful, stop-smoking shots were used as described in Chapter 12. This combined approach was successful with about 50 percent of the patients who previously had been classified as failures.

These are our results after three months. The long-term effects of the Stop-Smoking, Lose-Weight Diet and stop-smoking shots can be determined only through additional studies. However, there have been some responses from a number of my patients that you might find illuminating.

The patients who wrote me about failure of the shots to help them quit smoking were disappointed. Although they were upset at the lack of success, a minority did say they lacked the willpower to continue to try to kick their nicotine habit.

The comments from my patients that follow came unsolicited. I am grateful that they shared their experiences, both the good and the bad. The statements here are reprinted exactly as they came to my office, including the punctuation and underlining.

Some patients who were only partially successful in their stop-smoking efforts after having had the shots indicated that even some improvement is appreciated.

"I've only smoked a few cigarettes," wrote one patient. "Don't think I'll ever smoke regularly again. Thanks!"

Another confessed that, although smoking again, "rather than two to three packs a day, I can get by with five to ten cigarettes per day."

And a third who didn't break down and smoke a cigarette until three or four weeks after receiving the shots seemed very pleased at "smoking only one a day, four or five days a week."

Although the shots do not assist all patients to stop smoking, in many cases they have had a beneficial effect on their smoking habits.

Though one lady began smoking again six weeks after her shots, she nevertheless wrote us, happily, "My cluster headaches disappeared after five years of suffering daily. . . . Because of the shots, I learned that smoking triggers my headaches, so, hopefully, I will never smoke more than ten or fifteen a day, as the headaches return then."

I am particularly pleased with the positive responses received from patients who stopped smoking completely after having had the shots.

"Hope the Good Powers that be have heard me when I mention you and your staff in my prayers each night. Good luck and God bless."

And another gratifying response: "It was exactly as you

said. No *physical desire.* Tremendous psychological desire? *I am deeply grateful.* It worked! I have never felt better." (Underlining was the patient's.)

On the other hand, some of my patients seem surprised over the fact that they could quit completely.

A patient, matter-of-factly: "No preoccupation with the fact I stopped. Feel like I have always been a nonsmoker."

Complete cessation was particularly gratifying to this patient who gloated:

"After thirty-seven years of smoking without stopping, this method was most successful. It made it so very easy for me! This was the only reason I have quit. I had tried other methods and nothing else was successful."

It should be encouraging to anyone trying to give up cigarettes to read excerpts such as these from a few of my patients who received the stop-smoking injections.

The following is from a gentleman who "fell away" and did smoke again after only three weeks of abstinence. But, read for yourself:

"Since the date of treatment, I have smoked exactly four cigarettes, and now the urge (mental) is gone! These were smoked under stress conditions, at work, only. They were smoked one cigarette on one day, etc. . . . never more than one in a twenty-four-hour period.

"Repeat . . . now all urges seem to be gone. I *had* a two-pack-a-day habit of forty years' duration! I have gained *no* weight!!!"

And others:

"Complete success. Very slight desire for a cigarette now and then but, no hang-up after four months."

"After smoking continually for thirty-nine years, an average of three packs a day in later years, I stopped immediately after the treatment. Prior to Dr. Solomon's treatment, I tried everything, including hypnosis, but all to no avail."

"I've smoked for thirty years—tried to quit for twenty years. I finally did it. Thanks."

"I believe my ability to breathe has greatly improved."

14 • Slimming Tips

If you are trying to lose weight and stop smoking at the same time, exercise should be an integral part of your regime—along with the Stop-Smoking, Lose-Weight Diet. You will lose weight easier and healthier that way. Think of exercise and diet as partners.

Although exercise is an important adjunct to the Stop-Smoking, Lose-Weight Diet, I am not suggesting that it is necessary to become a trained athlete capable of running a marathon or swimming the English Channel. What I am discussing here is exercise in moderation—exercise that will not only aid in weight reduction but will improve your circulation and physical fitness as well.

WHY EXERCISE?

The following are my clinical impressions about exercise:

- Exercise helps you lose weight, stay slim, and increase your blood circulation. Endurance or aerobic exercises like jogging or running, vigorous swimming, or aerobic dancing, can burn off 350 to 600 calories an hour. And for up to six hours following a workout, you will continue to burn up calories at a higher rate than if you had remained inactive!

- Remember, obesity results when your caloric intake is greater than your caloric expenditure. A proper diet will lower your caloric intake. Regular exercise will boost your expenditure of energy and make it ever so much easier to lose weight.

- For those not seriously overweight, exercise can provide greater freedom in the selection of foods without creating concern about the possibility of putting on weight.

- Exercise can act as an appetite depressant. As you exercise, fat is broken down into keto-acids and released into your bloodstream. It acts on the hypothalamus as a built-in appetite depressant.

- Exercise can increase your strength and flexibility.

- As you increase your fitness, your heart gets stronger and more efficient. Each beat does more work, so your pulse at rest is lower than it was when you were out of condition. Your blood pressure eases down to a lower, more healthful level. Your body, including your heart, uses oxygen more effectively.

- Exercise promotes better circulation. It conditions your heart and lungs and improves your ability to take in increased amounts of oxygen and enrich your blood supply to your muscles and vital organs.

- People who exercise regularly tend to have less heart trouble. One especially revealing survey involved thousands of Harvard University graduates. The findings showed that the more vigorously and regularly they exercised, the smaller their chances of having a heart attack. The risk was only half as great in those expending 2,000 calories in exercise per week (the equivalent of running a total of twenty miles at eight minutes per mile) as in those who expended less than 500 calories.

- Vigorous exercise may reduce a fatty substance in the blood called triglycerides, which can be a risk if their level is too high. And in a fit body, the blood has less tendency to clot, so there is less chance of a blockage that may cause a stroke or heart attack.

- Exercise can have a dramatic impact on blood cholesterol—an important factor in cardiovascular health. The change in *total* cholesterol is not very marked (although it is somewhat lower in those who exercise regularly and strenuously). The big difference is in the balance between high-density lipoprotein (HDL) and low-density lipoprotein (LDL). Dr. Peter D. Ward and his colleagues at Stanford University found that the beneficial HDL was about 50 percent higher in people who exercised strenuously. Even for those who exercised only moderately, there was a very significant shift from the harmful LDL to the helpful HDL.

- Exercise makes you look better. It tones and shapes your body. Even your complexion is improved.

- Exercise can release your tensions, lift your spirit, and improve your attitude. After a busy day trying to cope with life's stresses, what better way to relax than a period of exercise? And since the way we feel about ourselves is linked to the way we look, as our bodies change for the better so does our attitude about ourselves.

- And finally, regular exercise can enhance your sex life!

In my last book, *Dr. Solomon's High Health Diet & Exercise Plan*, I discuss the three kinds of exercises ideally you should do. All three kinds are incorporated in the exercises prepared for you in this chapter. Furthermore, I have used information from my previous book which I thought would be helpful to you in doing the exercises.

First, there is exercise that makes and keeps you limber, that prevents muscles from shortening, that maintains the fullest range of joint movement. An example is touching your toes. This kind is usually called *stretching* or *flexibility* exercise.

Then there is *strengthening* exercise, which builds up the power of various skeletal muscles. Push-ups are a good example.

Last, but definitely not least, is exercise that conditions your heart-lung system—*endurance* or *aerobic* exercise. This improves your ability to take in oxygen. Your heart pumps it all around your body and uses it in the production of energy.

Endurance exercise is the most important. It is the only way to get your cardiovascular system in good condition. It requires using the big muscles of your body in a steady, rhythmical way so that you raise your heartbeat and your rate of breathing. Fast walking, jogging or running, vigorous swimming, cross-country skiing, rowing, aerobic dancing, and jazz exercise are excellent. So are sports like squash and racquet ball. And tennis, if you really keep going.

To be effective, endurance activity has to be done continuously over a period of time. A sensible minimum to shoot for is twenty minutes, three times a week. Of course, if you are out of shape you will have to build up to this gradually. Let your body be your guide.

HOW OFTEN?

It is best to make exercise a daily habit, but if you can't manage this, try to get in at least three periods of endurance exercise a week, and an equal number of stretching and strengthening sessions.

A little perseverance may be necessary at first. But once you start realizing the benefits of regular exercise—that it makes you look and feel better—chances are you will be hooked on exercise as a way of life.

BEFORE STARTING— A MEDICAL CHECK-UP

It is a good idea to check with your doctor before launching into an exercise program. If you are in your twenties or early thirties, in pretty good condition, and have never had any serious medical problem, you may not need a physical examination. But one is certainly advisable if you are over thirty-five and have not been very active recently.

If you have—or have had—any problem, such as heart trouble, you should be sure to consult your doctor before starting, no matter what your age. That does not mean vigorous exercise is ruled out—in fact, exercise is now used routinely in the rehabilitation of people who have had heart attacks; some of them, after a long and very gradual buildup, have even gone on to marathon running. But you should follow a program that has your doctor's approval.

START SLOWLY

If you have not been doing much besides getting to the office or driving to the shopping center, be sure to start your exercise program slowly and increase it gradually over the weeks and months.

I find that often the simplest and most practical way to get sedentary patients started is plain walking. For others, I recommend a group exercise program where patients exercise under the direction of trained staff and where group reinforcement gives them the encouragement they need.

In any event, don't push yourself beyond your capacity. If you do, especially if you've been inactive for some time, you'll become discouraged and lose interest. Start slowly—build up gradually. Let your body be your guide.

IF YOUR BODY PROTESTS

You may be a little stiff at first. Any muscle discomfort can best be treated by simply repeating the limbering-up and stretching exercise. Soaking in a warm tub also helps to ease soreness.

WARNING SIGNS AND WHAT TO DO

When you take up systematic exercise, know your warning signs. If any of the following happens during or after exercising, stop your program and check with your doctor before resuming—immediately if the symptoms persist at all.

- Pain in the chest or radiating into the throat or arms. This is not necessarily a sign of heart trouble, but it could be. Regardless of exercise, if you ever have these symptoms for more than a minute or two, call for emergency medical services and get to a hospital emergency room.
- Irregular heartbeats—palpitations or a series of abnormally fast or slow beats. These kinds of irregularities can be harmless. Or they may require medical attention. Continued fast pulse five or ten minutes after exercising may mean you have been pushing yourself too hard.
- Dizziness, cold sweat, confusion. This probably means your brain is not getting enough blood. First aid: Lie down and put your feet up.

Some other points:

- Nausea after exercise, prolonged fatigue, or insomnia, indicates you are exercising too vigorously.
- If you have any arthritic or other joint problems that flare up, you may know from past experience how to deal with them. If they persist or get worse, check with your doctor.
- Shin splints and other muscular aches and pains are very often helped by wearing shoes with thicker soles. If necessary, shift to another exercise–for example, biking instead of jogging–until the ailment clears up.

P.S. Don't let any of these cautions scare you off from a good exercise regimen. Just bear them in mind to avoid getting into trouble.

WHAT THE MEN ARE MISSING

Recently, I attended a fascinating demonstration of aerobic dancing conducted by Lynn Rosen and Bette-Lynn Steiner at the Body Workshop, Inc., in Baltimore.

The program contains a number of special features that make it especially attractive to my patients:

- It combines flexibility, strength, and endurance exercises.
- Aerobic routines are designed to be high-calorie burners while slimming and trimming legs, hips, and stomach.
- The program strengthens the heart and lungs and increases circulation, especially to the extremities. Since smokers often experience numbness in their extremities as the result of poor circulation, this program can literally "put them in touch" with their own bodies again.
- You participate at your own level of fitness and skill.
- The heart rate is monitored regularly to determine stress.
- Best of all—it's fun to do!

GETTING STARTED

What to Wear

Wear loose-fitting clothing so that you can move and breathe freely—for example, T-shirts and shorts, warm-up suits, or leotards and tights.

Athletic shoes are a must. These should be tennis shoes, not jogging shoes, to allow for forward-backward, as well as side-to-side movement. Shoes should have good heel support and heel cushioning. Wear sport socks. It is important not to jog-dance on the balls of your feet.

Breathing

Correct breathing is important to your feeling of well-being. It can calm and relax you, clean excessive amounts of carbon dioxide out of the blood, increase your circulation, and give you a natural high.

Relaxercizers

Slow, controlled movements along with soothing music help my patients attain a sense of relaxation, revitalize them, and increase their capacity to deal with stress—including the stress of not having a cigarette.

Here are two breathing exercises that can help you:

Breathing Exercise Number 1

Sit with legs in a "V" and arms overhead. Tuck tummy in tight and breathe in through your nose. Then release the air through your mouth as you let your tummy out and bend forward at the waist. Repeat five times.

Breathing Exercise Number 2

Stand with your arms at your side. Breathe in through your nose as you raise your arms over your head. Release air through your mouth as your arms are lowered and your knees are bent.

Music, Music, Music

The aerobic dance program is designed to be easy to follow and you will have fun doing it! Add a little music and get into the beat. Add your own style and make your movements dancelike. Pretend you are on stage or in the boxing ring. Fantasize a little and select music that fits your mood. By doing this, you will subconsciously be disguising your hard work, and the time spent exercising will be fun, enjoyable, and exciting.

For the warm-up and the cool-down, select music with a slower beat. Many numbers by Barbra Streisand and Barry Manilow are especially good for this purpose.

For the aerobic portion, switch to something more upbeat—disco, Broadway, pop, etc. You can have a lot of fun doing your own thing.

The Warm-Up

Any endurance workout should be preceded by a brief warm-up—at least five minutes—and followed by a cool-down of the same length. You can work some limbering exercises into these periods and two or three strengthening exercises if you like.

The warm-up has several purposes. It gets your muscles and joints ready for the vigorous exercise that lies ahead. A "cold" muscle is not as supple as a warm one, and therefore is more easily injured. Also, it is advisable to increase your heartbeat gradually since a sudden load placed on it might be dangerous for a person not in good physical condition.

The warm-up exercises are specifically designed to prepare the body for an aerobic workout.

Remember:

- Don't rush. Take minibreaks—especially if you are just starting.

- Avoid jerky movements.

- Don't force yourself. Don't try to rush ahead. Don't compete with other people or with what you did yesterday.

- If you do not have a good mat, avoid kneeling or rolling-on-your-back exercises.

I hope I have been able to convince you that exercise can be fun. Fortunately, more and more Americans are reaching this conclusion and are becoming more active every day. Unfortunately, far too many Americans are still overweight and underactive.

According to the Food and Nutrition Board of the National Research Council, approximately 30 percent of middle-aged women and 15 percent of middle-aged men in the United States are obese—that is, more than 120 percent of their ideal weight.

Everyone wants to live longer, but the quality of life is also important. Keeping fit is the key. Most of us can achieve this goal by controlling our food intake and exercising, and by not abusing our bodies with such harmful habits as smoking.

But it does take commitment. Bad habits are not easy to break. I have tried to point you on the path to good health. You must supply the motivation, self-discipline, and patience to follow it.

I know you can do it!

TIME FOR AEROBICS

Before you begin, put on your favorite upbeat music and try the recommended steps in front of a mirror. If it helps, hold the book in front of you.
- Don't get bogged down in trying to learn all the steps at once.
- When a few of the steps are familiar, put them together and then start the music.
- Begin with three 10 to 15 minute sessions a week. Work up gradually until you can comfortably handle 20 to 30 minutes at a stretch.

REMEMBER:
- If you are really out of shape, give yourself time to get into condition.
- Whenever you jump, be sure to land with slightly bent knees and flat on your feet to absorb the shock.

If you like, try putting two steps together to match the beat of your favorite music, and dance to the beat of the song. This motivates you and lifts your mood! Turn on the radio or stereo and exercise away!

Here are some possible routines:

8 Punch-Jog
8 Side Jumps
Hip 2, Jog 4
Rocky 8
8 Whippers
4 Clap-Downs
4 Knee-Lifts
2 Knee Twists, Clap 2
Jump Jog 4
Flick Kick 8
Routines can be repeated as often as enjoyable.

THE COOL-DOWN

The cool-down is also important. If you stop abruptly after strenuous exercise, the blood that has been coursing through your muscles slows down and may be trapped for a moment. As a result, your brain may not get enough and you will feel faint or dizzy. Or your heart muscle will not get sufficient blood, in which case you may notice some extra heartbeats. If your intestines are deprived of blood, you will probably feel nauseated.

The cool-down enables you to reduce your blood pressure and pulse rate smoothly and gradually. You may have noticed athletes cooling down with slow jogging or walking, or horses being walked after a race. It is important to follow their example.

The following cool-down exercises and relaxercisers are recommended by the Body Workshop.

WARM-UP EXERCISES

#1 *"Calf Stretches"—to stretch calf muscles*

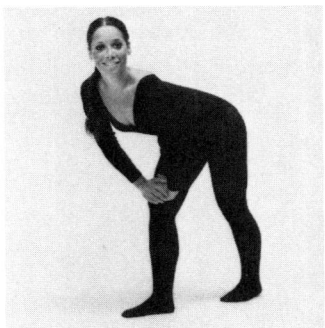

Stand. Place one leg three feet in front of the other. Bend the front leg, placing your weight on it. Both feet are flat on the floor and facing straight ahead. Place hands on front knee and hold for a count of ten. Repeat on the opposite leg.

#2 *"Jazz Twister"—for the waist*

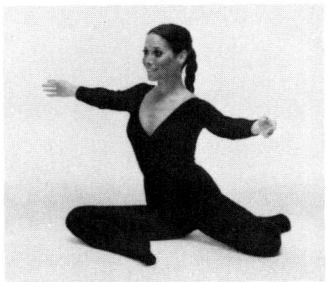

Sit on floor with one leg in front of the other. Arms open out to sides.

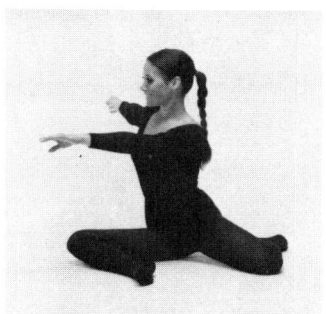

Twist from waist up as far right as possible, keeping hips and legs still.

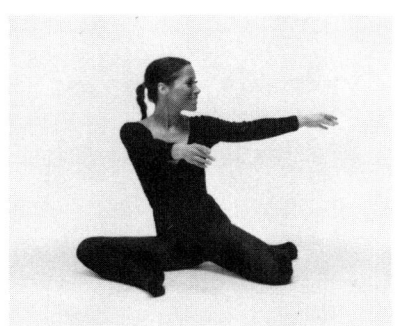

Twist left.

#3 "Heel Taps"—for the thighs and calfs

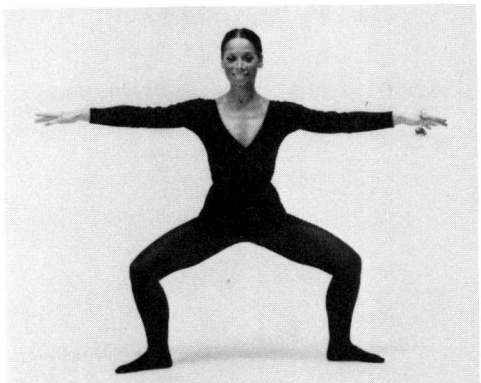

Stand with feet about three feet apart, toes pointing outward. Arms out to side. Bend knees as low as possible. torso remains immobile.

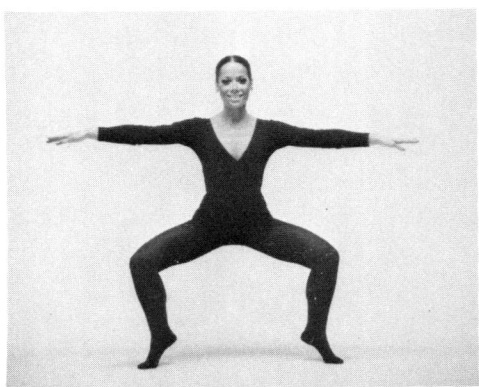

Lift and lower heels as high as possible to the beat of the music. Repeat 20 times.

#4 "Hand Shakes"—for circulation

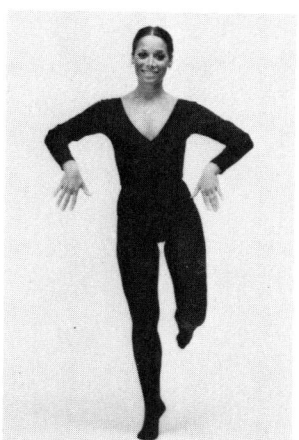

While jogging in place, shake both hands twice in front of your body to the beat of the music.

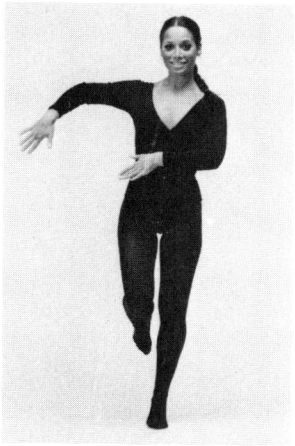

Shake both hands twice to the right.

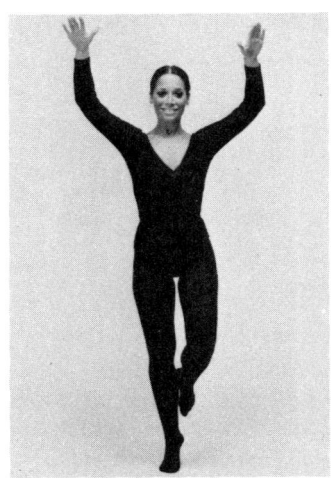

Shake both hands overhead twice.

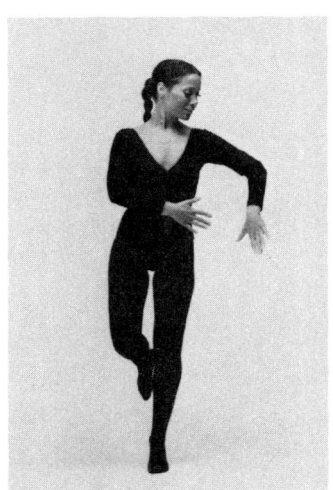

Shake both hands twice to the left of body. (Keep jogging during this exercise)

#5 "Torso Slide"—for the waist

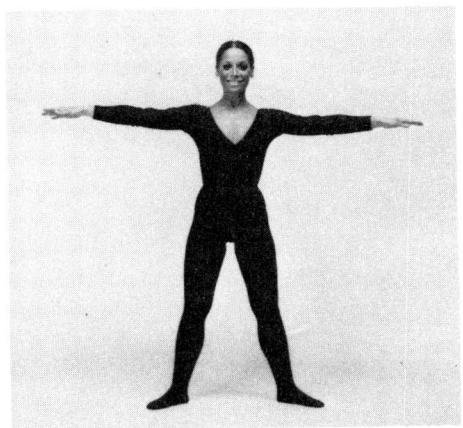

Stand . . . arms open to sides . . . feet about three feet apart.

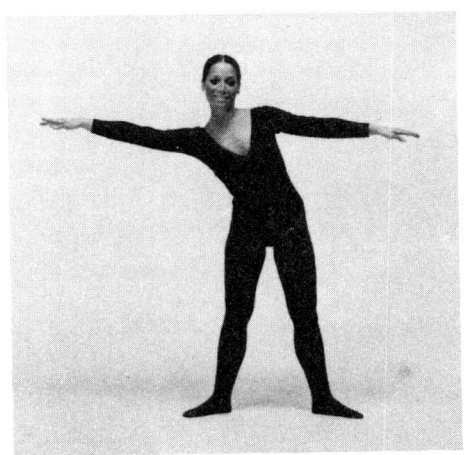

Slide upper body from waist up as far over to right as possible.

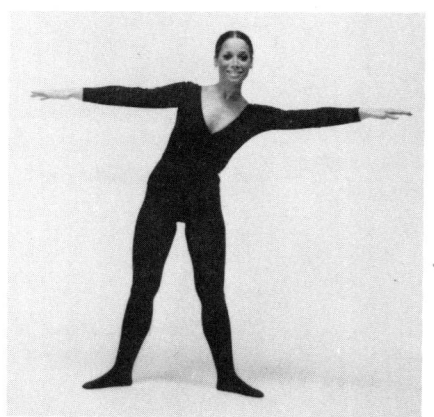

Then slide upper body as far over to left as possible. Repeat exercise 20 times. Remember to keep hips immobile during entire exercise.

#6 *"Hip Circles"—circulation and waist*

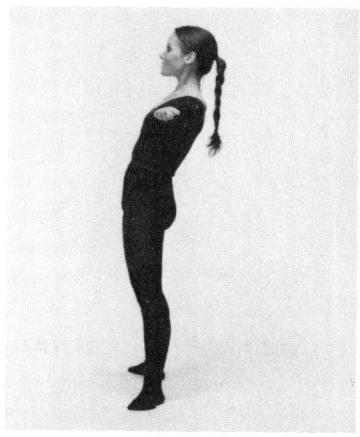

Stand with feet about one foot apart. Push hips forward.

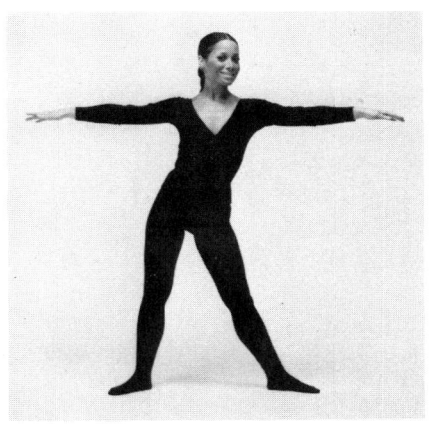

Then rotate hips to right side.

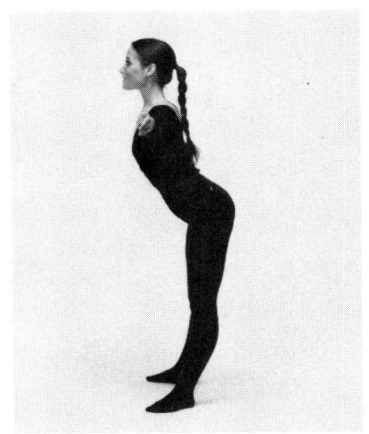

Rotate hips to rear.

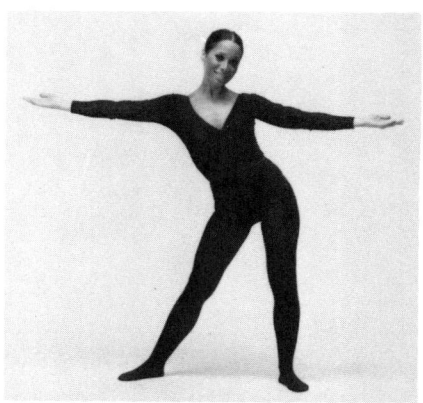

Rotate hips to left side. This exercise should be done fluidly and nonstop. Keep legs straight. Repeat 10 times in each direction.

#7 *"Shoulder Shimmy"—for circulation*

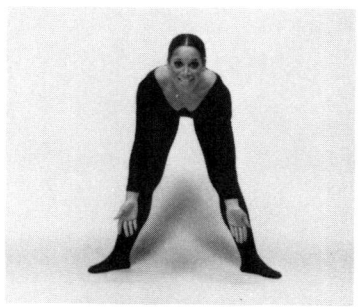

Stand. Bend over at the waist. Let your arms hang down.

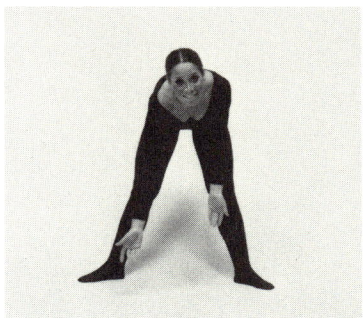

Let your right shoulder drop down, then your left. Alternate back and forth until you have a fast shimmy.

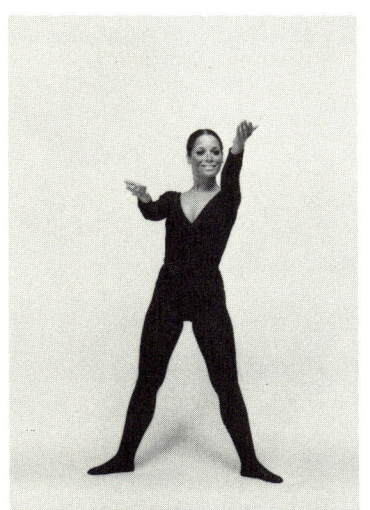
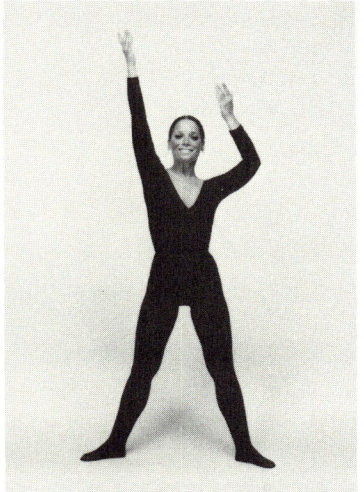

Then shimmy on up to a standing position with your arms moving slowly up until they are over your head. Do for one minute.

#8 "Hip Swivels"—for underthighs, abdominal muscles, and derriere

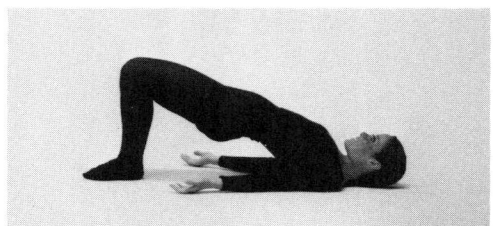

Lie on your back on the floor, hands by your sides. Bend your knees and place your feet flat on the floor. Lift your hips up as level to your knees as possible. Try to keep your knees together.

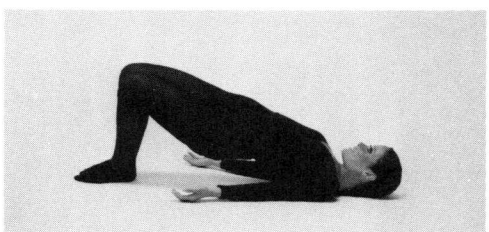

Rotate your right hip to the ceiling, then rotate your left hip to the ceiling. Keep doing this alternating each hip until you have a faster swivel. Try not to lower hips below knee level during this exercise. 30 times.

#9 "The Bender"—waist slimmer

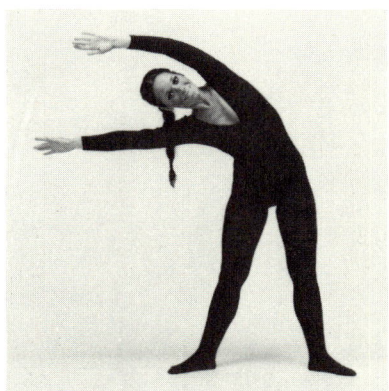

Stand with your feet apart and your arms open to the sides. Bring your left arm over your head and to the right side as you dip your upper body, from the waist up, to your right for two bounces.

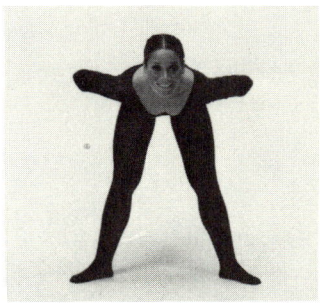

Then, with your hands on your waist and your chin up, bounce forward twice.

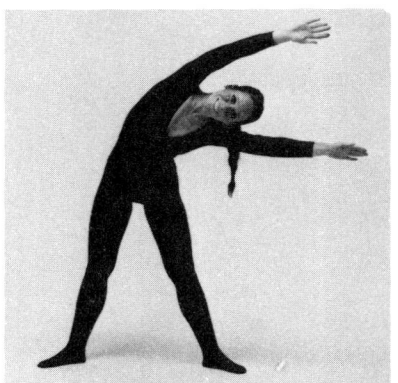

Now bring your right arm over to the left side and bounce twice. Repeat this sequence 8 times.

#10 "Leg Straddles"—leg stretches

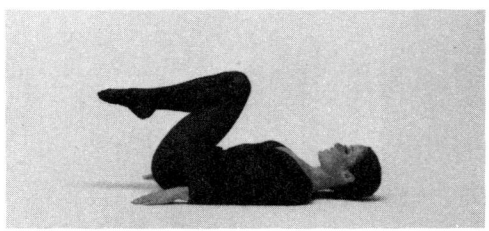

Lie on your back on the floor. Bring your knees up to your chest.

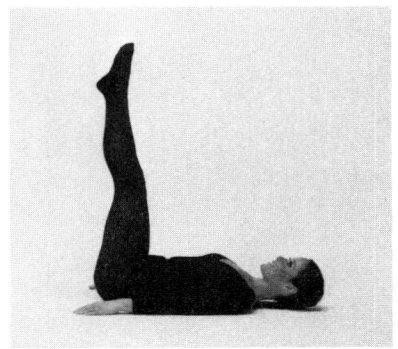

Lift both legs straight up.

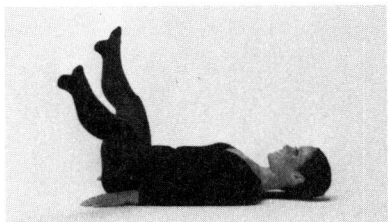

Open wide slowly into a "V" position. Bring legs together as in first step and repeat.

#11 "Roundabouts"—abdominal strengthener

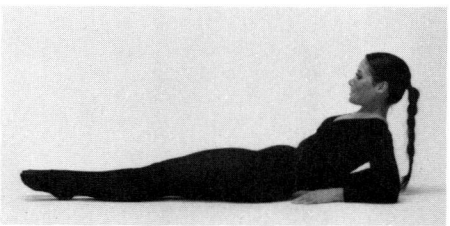

Lie on your back, resting on your elbows.

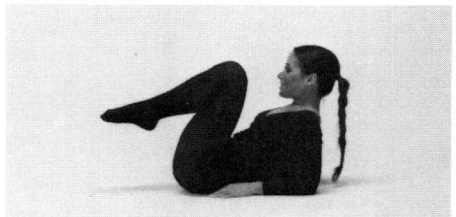

Bring both knees up to your chest.

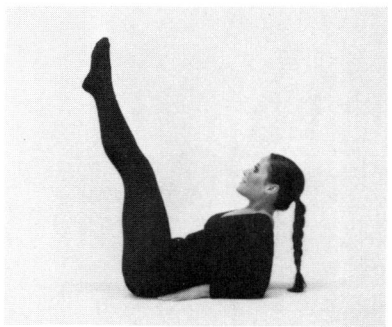

Bring legs straight up.

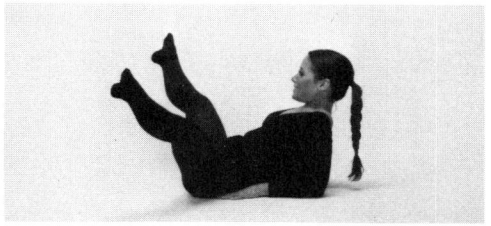

Open your legs slowly into a wide "V" position.

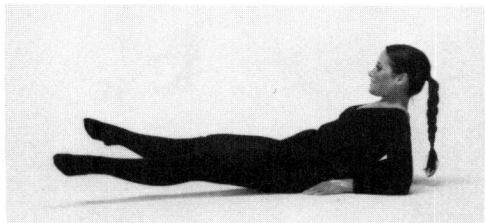

Continue to bring legs around in front of you, keeping them inches off the floor.

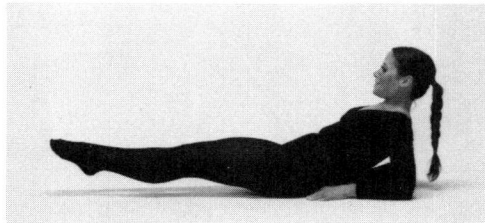

Finish in this position. This is done in a low, parallel, and circular motion. Repeat 10 times.

#12 "Arm Scissors"—circulation and arm strengthener

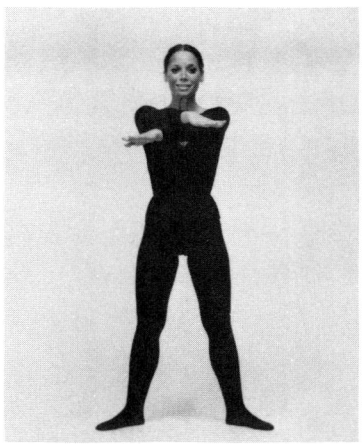

Stand, feet apart. Cross arms in front of your chest at shoulder level. Cross right arm over left, then left arm over right. Do this rapidly.

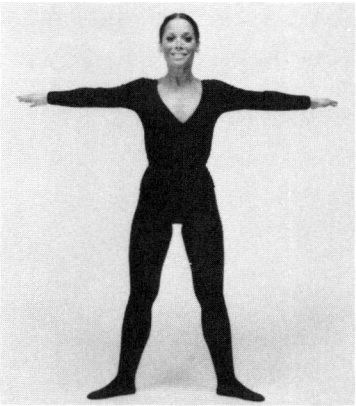

Then open arms wide to sides, bouncing them back twice. Keep arms at shoulder level. Repeat 10 times.

AEROBIC EXERCISES

#1 "Flasher"—calf-strengthener, circulation

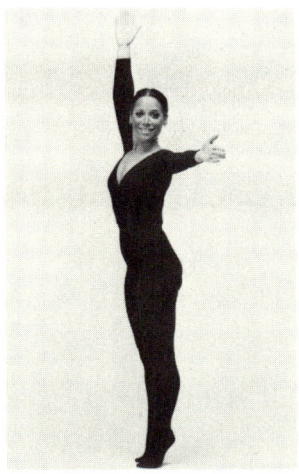

Arms at sides. Jump up onto the balls of your feet. Raise arms in an "L" when you jump, left arm extended, right arm above head.

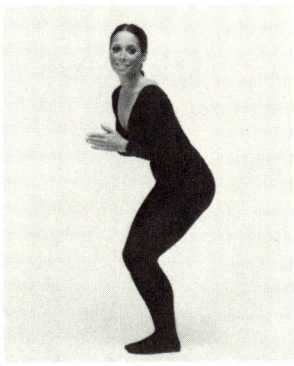

Jump back down, knees bent, feet flat on floor. Clap your hands.

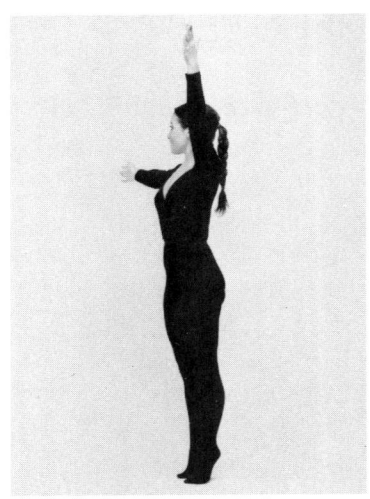

Repeat first step but right arm extended, left arm above head.

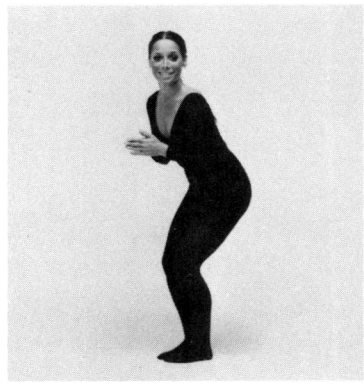

Repeat second step (jump back down) 10 times.

#2 "Flick-Kick"—thigh slimmer, circulation

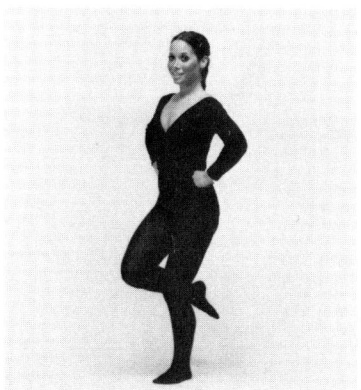

Stand on your left foot and bend your right leg back at the knee.

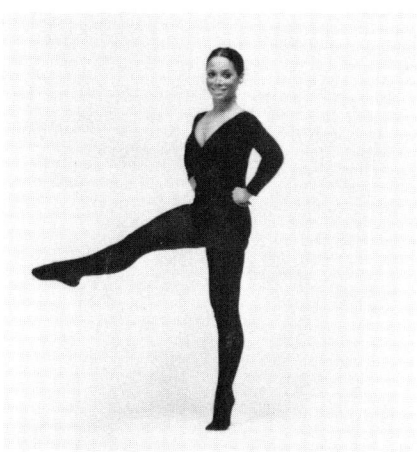

Kick right leg straight out. When you have the movement, add a hop. Alternate legs. 10 times on each leg.

#3 "Whipper"

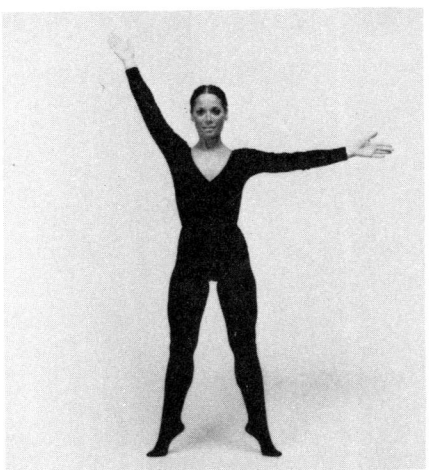

Stand with your feet apart and toes turned out. Jump up onto the balls of your feet.

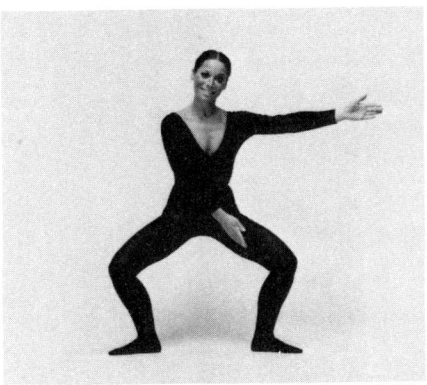

Jump back down onto a full foot, making sure that both knees are bent—the lower the better. Arms make a whipping motion. Repeat 10 times to one side, then 10 times to the other side.

#4 "Hip 2, Jog 4"—circulation

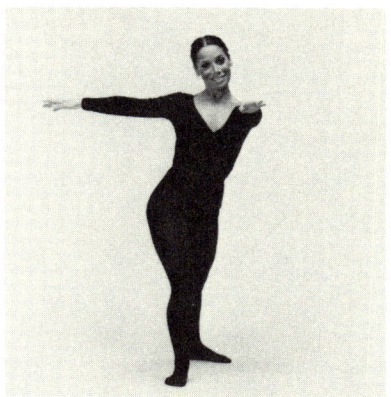

Push your right hip over your right foot as you step forward onto it.

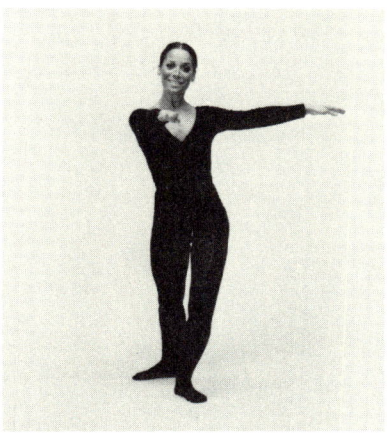

Your left foot then steps forward as you push your left hip over it.

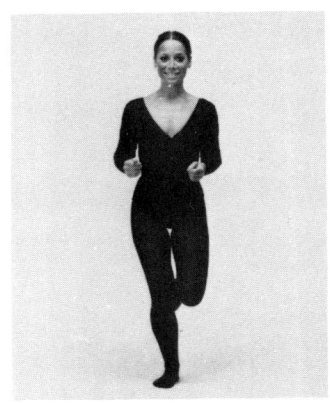

Then jog in place 4 times. Repeat 10 times.

#5 *"Knee Twist, Clap 2"—waist slimmer, circulation*

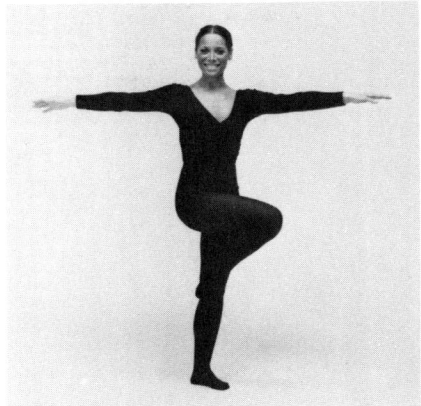

Bring your right foot up alongside your left knee. Hop as you swivel your right knee toward your left hip.

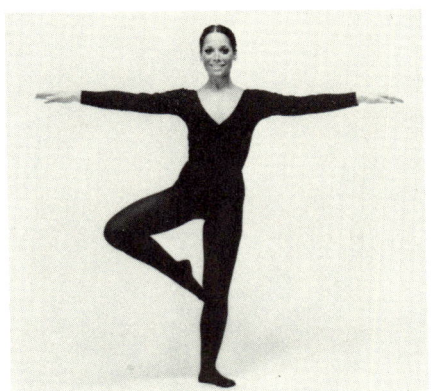

Then hop again as you swivel your knee back to the starting position.

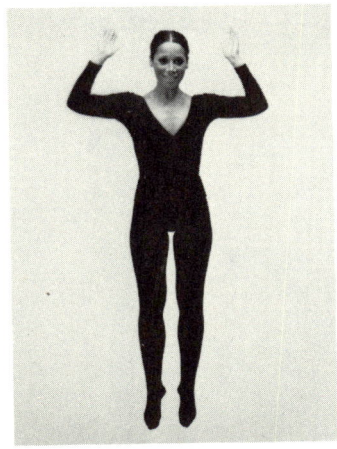

Jump with feet together twice as you clap twice. Repeat 10 times on each leg.

#6 "Knee Lifts"—leg strengthener, circulation

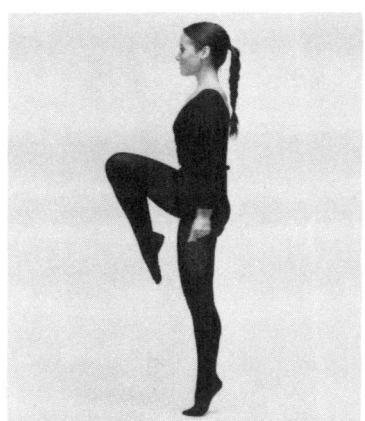

Lift your right knee as high as you can. Once you have the movement, add a jump to it. Each time your knee comes up, you jump to get it up. Snap your fingers to each lift. Repeat, alternating on each leg. 10 times on each leg.

#7 "Kick-Outs"—thigh slimmer, circulation, leg strengthener

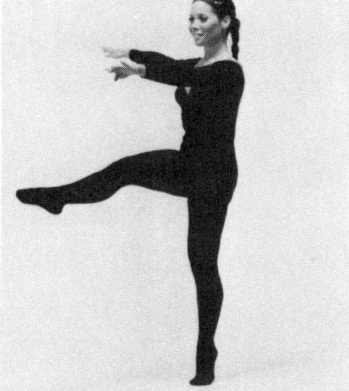

Kick your right leg straight ahead as you hop high on your left foot. Return to standing position and repeat with left leg. Travel forward on each kick-out. Whenever you hop up, come down on a slightly bent knee. 10 times each leg.

#8 "Crazy Jog"—for circulation and stamina

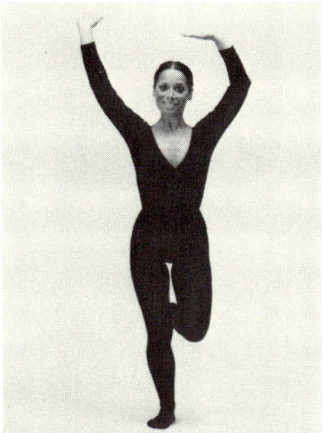

Jog in a wide circle, 16 counts with your arms over your head and palms to the ceiling. Wave your arms wildly to the music. Repeat circle left.

#9 "Jog 2, Hop 2"—calf strengthener, circulation

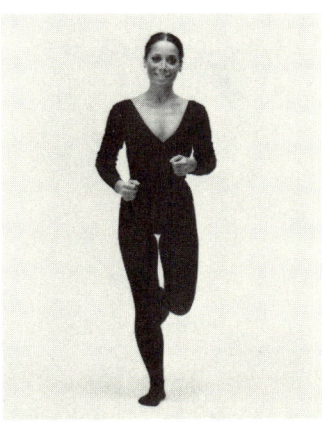

Jog right foot, left foot, then hop on right foot twice. Repeat the jog, hopping twice on left foot. Repeat sequence 10 times.

#10 "Jumper"—waist and upper torso trimmer, circulation

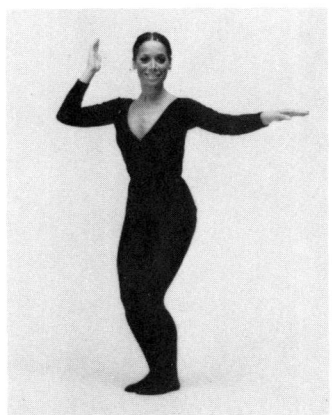

Feet are together. Jump 2 times slightly to the right.

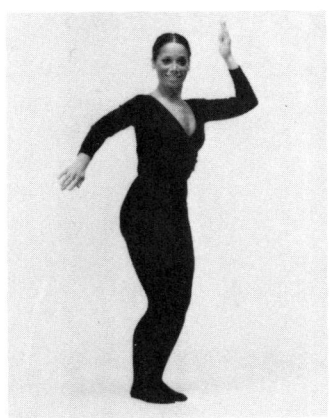

Then jump twice slightly to the left, jump 4 single jumps, rotating right, left, right, left. Repeat 4 times.

#11 "Jump Jog"—stamina, circulation

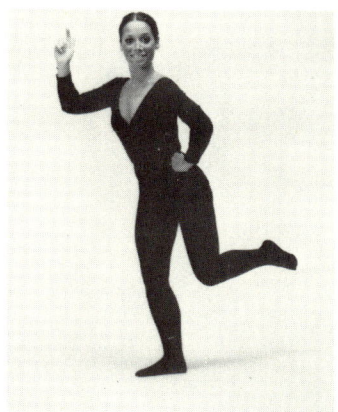

Left hand on your waist, right arm bent. Point with your finger. Hop forward onto your right foot.

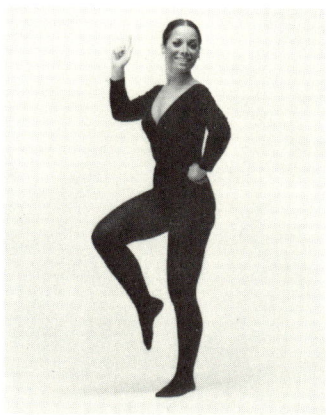

Then jog upright for 8 counts. Repeat 4 times.

#12 "Punch-Jog"

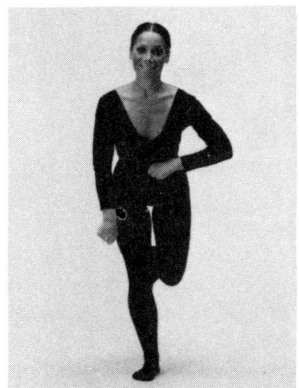

Jog in place as you punch, alternating right, left, and downward toward the floor.

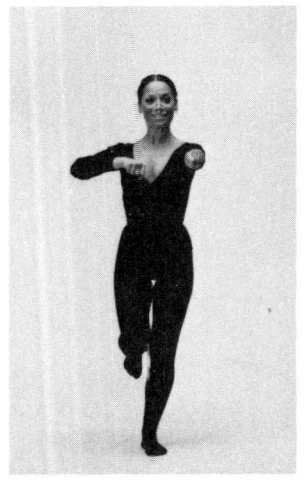

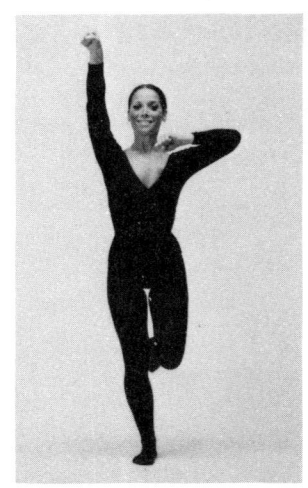

Then keep on punching as your arms move slowly up . . .

Until you are punching over your head.

#13 "Side Jumps"—circulation, stamina

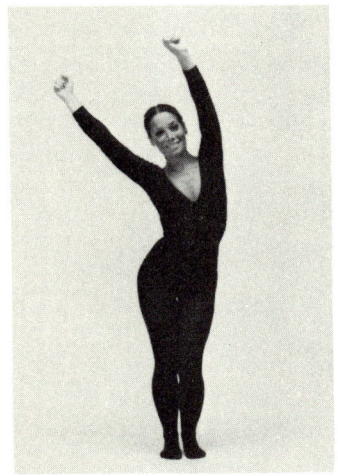

With your arms overhead and hands fisted . . .

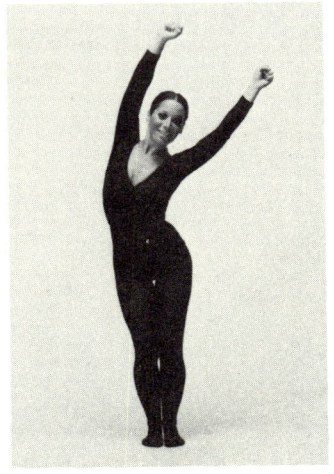

Jump with feet together from side to side. Arms move in same direction as body. Do 10 times.

#14 "Rocky"—circulation and thighs

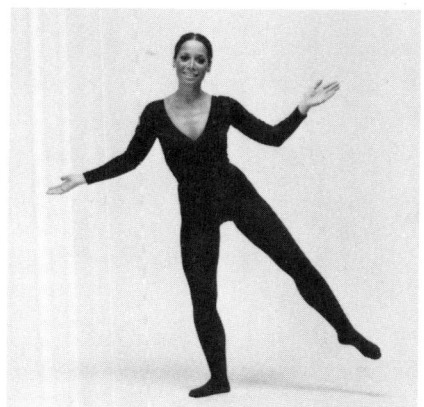

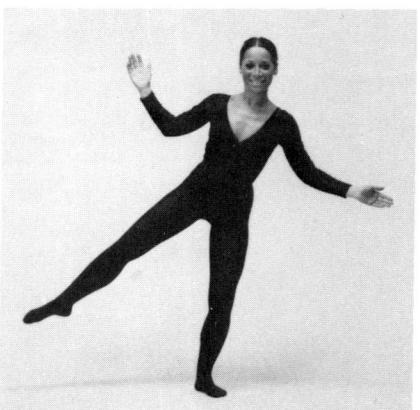

Hop on your right foot and at the same time extend your left leg low and out to the left side. Then hop onto your left foot and extend your right foot out to the right side at the same time. Rock back and forth from one side to the other like this, 10 times, alternating right, left, right, left. Arms outside, bent at elbow.

#15 "Freddy Flip"—circulation and thighs

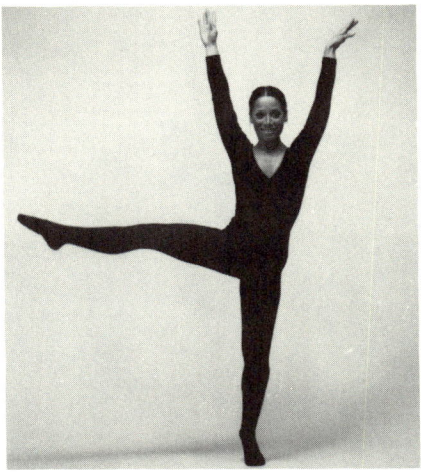

Bring your right leg up and out straight to the right side as high as possible. Arms fly overhead as you kick out to the side.

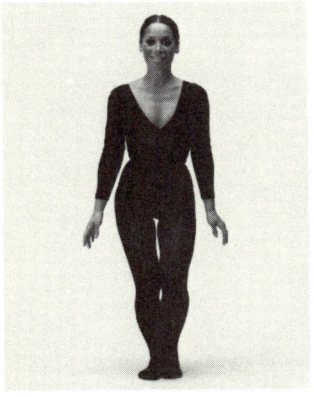

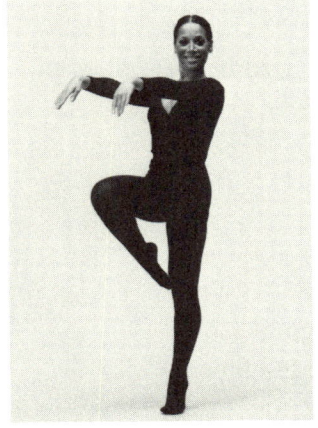

Then hop on your left foot as you bring it back down. Arms drop back down.

Hop again on your left foot as you bring your right knee up toward your chest. Flip your hands down as your knee comes up. Alternate on your other side. Do 6 times.

#16 "Front 2, Back 2"—circulation and stamina

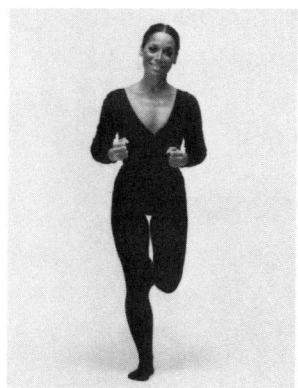

Jog forward for 2—right foot, left foot; jog back for 2—right foot, left foot. Always start on your right foot. Repeat four times.

#17 "Jump-Scissors"—circulation, leg trimmer, calfs and thighs, arm toner

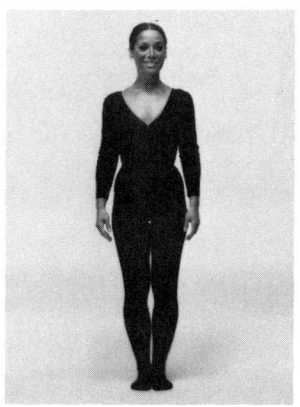

Stand with feet together.

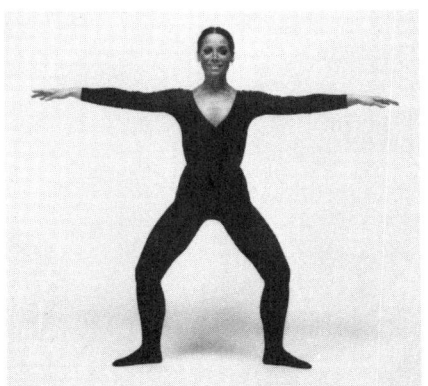

Jump with feet and arms apart. Land first with slightly bent knees.

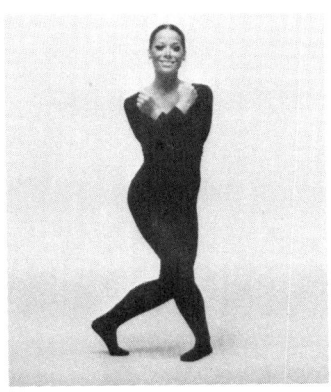

Then jump together as right leg crosses in front of left leg. Arms crossed in front of chest, hands fisted. Reverse arms and legs each time you jump together. Repeat 10 times.

#18 "Clap Down"—thighs, arms, stamina, circulation

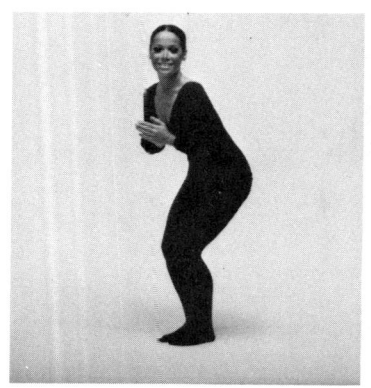 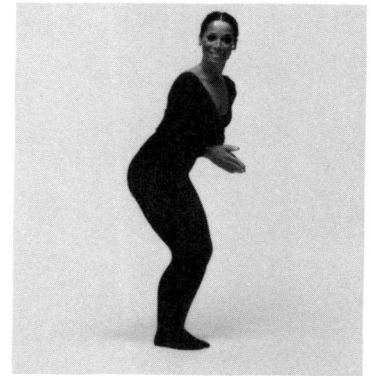

Clap as you jump right.　　　Clap as you jump left.

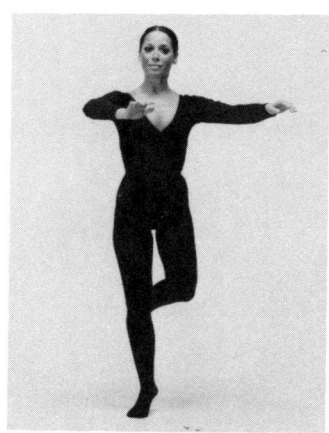

Run forward 4 counts. Repeat 6 times.

COOL-DOWN EXERCISES

#1 "Shin Bounces"—shins

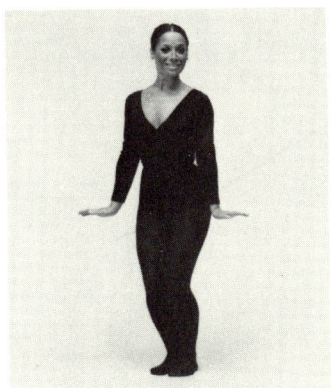

Feet together, flat on floor. Slowly bend knees directly over toes and hold for count 6. Repeat 4 times.

#2 "Shoulder Twists"—shoulders

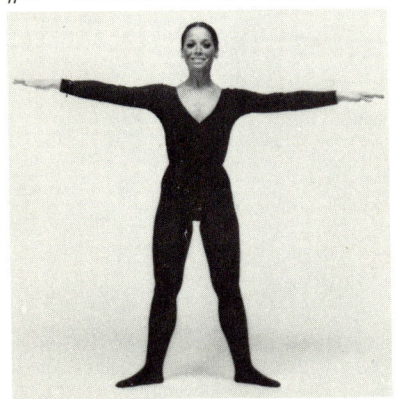
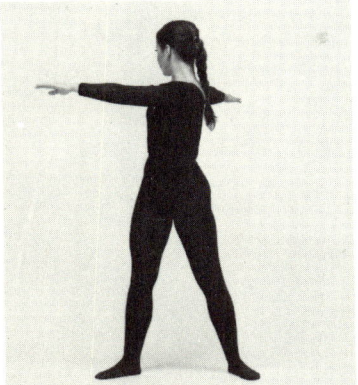

Arms extended. Twist from your waist up to the right, once, around as far back as comfortably possible. Repeat to the left side.

#3 "Waist Whittlers"—waist

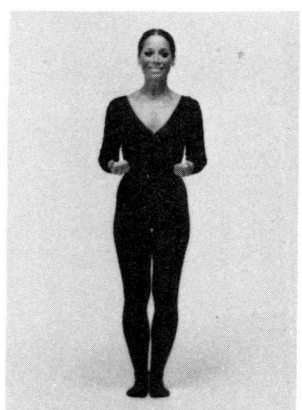

Arms bent, elbows against waist, hands fisted. Hips remain full front and immobile as you rotate from the waist up . . .

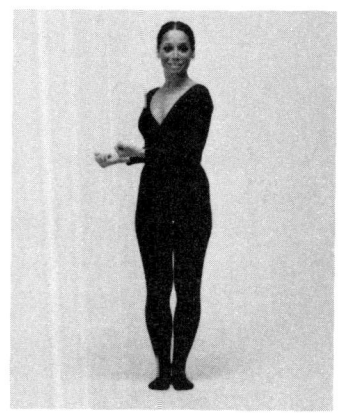

To the right . . .

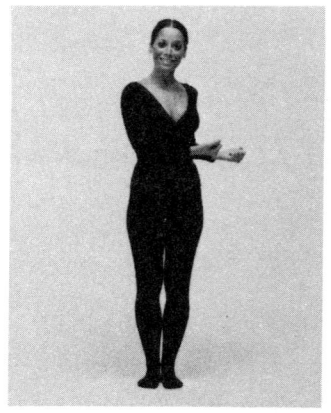

Then left. Swivel upper body at an increasing pace for one minute.

#4 "Fly-Away"—shoulders, circulation, relaxation

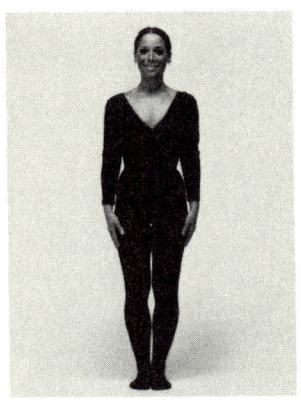

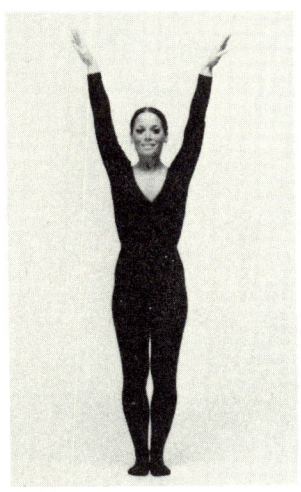

Arms at sides. As you breathe in through your nose, slowly bring arms over head. Breathe out through your mouth and slowly return arms to sides.

#5 "Cross Fly"—*stretching, circulation*

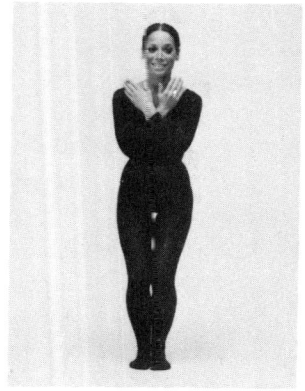

Feet together, knees slightly bent. Cross arms in front of chest.

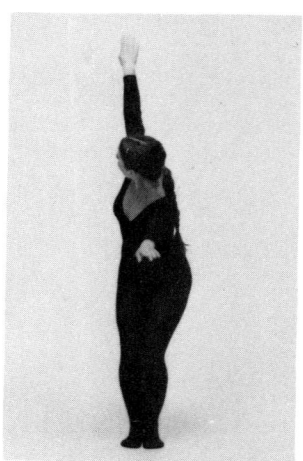

Twist upper torso to right, opening arms wide. Look up at right hand.

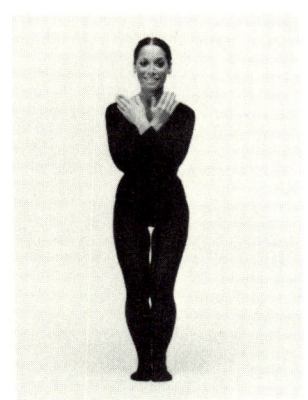

Feet together, knees slightly bent. Cross arms in front of chest.

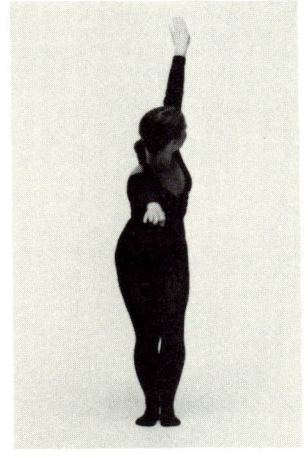

Twist upper torso left, opening arms wide. Look up at left hand. Repeat 8 times.

#6 "Sit Indian Style"—position for exercises numbers 6–14

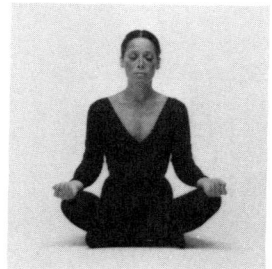

Sit cross-legged, with the backs of your hands resting on your knees, palms up. Eyes closed. All movements done in this position are done in slow motion—no jerky movements.

#7 "Chin Lifts"—chin toner; tension reducer

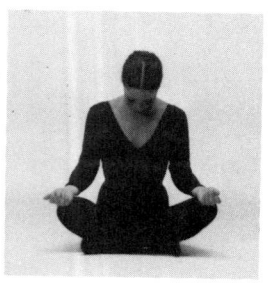 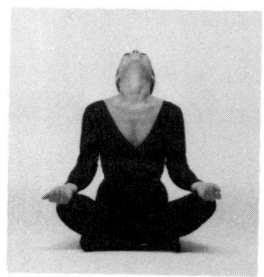

Sitting Indian style, slowly lower chin to chest and then up to the ceiling. Repeat 6 times.

#8 "Slow Head Rolls"—neck toner and tension reducer

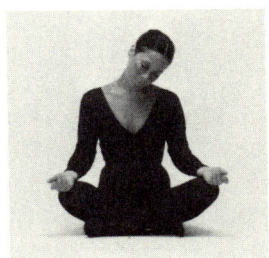

Sitting Indian style, lower your chin to your chest; roll head around in complete circle. Slowly let gravity take your head down and around. Repeat twice. Then change directions.

#9 "Slow No's"—neck toner and tension reducer

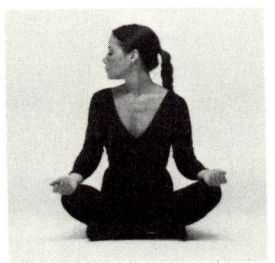

Sitting Indian style, slowly move your head in a "no" movement. Repeat 6 times.

#10 "Ear to Shoulder"—neck toner and tension release

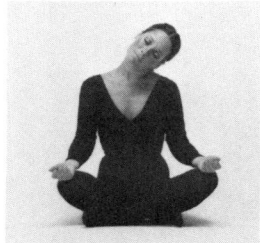

Sitting Indian style, bring your ear toward your shoulder slowly. Alternate sides. Repeat 6 times.

#11 "Arm Swims"—strengthens shoulders and releases tension

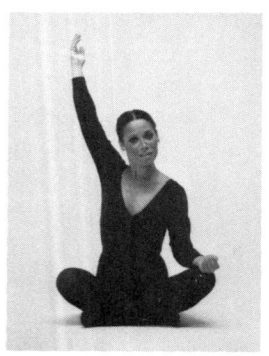 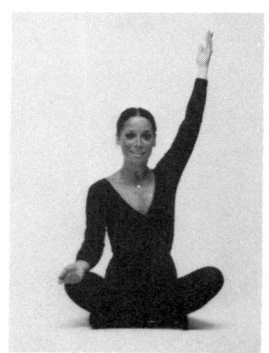

Sitting Indian style, do the swimmer's backstroke with your arms. Repeat 10 times, alternating arms.

Then alternate right, left, right, left. Repeat 4 times.

#12 "Shoulder Rolls"—releases shoulder-muscle tension

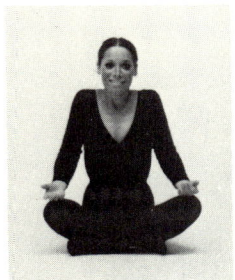 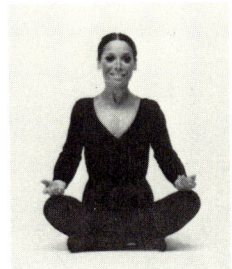 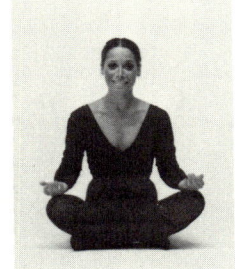

Sitting Indian style, slowly move both shoulders forward, up, back, and down. Repeat entire roll 4 times at a slow pace.

#13 "Silent Alphabet"—facial and neck toner, tension reducer.

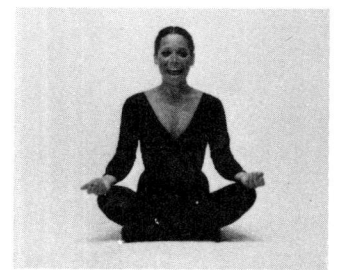 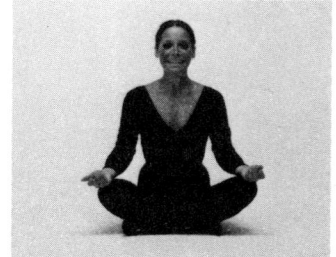

Sitting Indian style, silently and slowly say your ABCs, using your mouth in its widest movements. Exaggerate each letter. Use your whole face.

#14 "Kiss to Good Health!"—cheek and neck toner, tension reducer

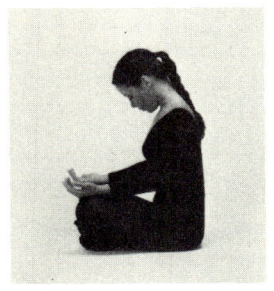

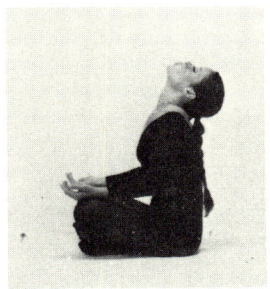

Sitting Indian style, bring your chin to your chest and slowly lift your chin to the ceiling as you pucker up and throw a big kiss. Repeat 4 times.

Afterword

I'm not claiming that my regimen is a panacea for everyone. I feel strongly that I am offering a common sense, medically based approach to alleviate the most common complaints that have been expressed by my nicotine-addicted patients.

In trying to help them, in helping them, with all the interest, empathy, and medical knowledge that I have gained over the past two decades, I hope I have helped you too.

If you smoke, are or are not overweight, and want to kick the habit, why not start now on my Stop-Smoking, Lose-Weight Diet? I would also appreciate knowing how successful you were. Please write and tell me, and add any helpful tips that I can pass on.

Thank you.

Neil Solomon, M.D., Ph.D.
1726 Reisterstown Road
Baltimore, Maryland 21208

NEIL SOLOMON, M.D., Ph.D.

Current and/or Past Medical School Faculty Positions

Assistant Professor, the Johns Hopkins University School of Medicine

Clinical Professor, University of Miami School of Medicine

Assistant Professor of Medicine, University of Maryland School of Medicine

Associate Professor of Physiology, University of Maryland School of Medicine